CHEN STYLE TAIJIQUAN

The Source of Taiji Boxing

CHEN STYLE TAIJIQUAN

The Source of Taiji Boxing

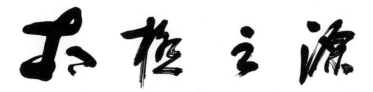

Davidine Siaw-Voon Sim
&
David Gaffney

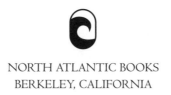

NORTH ATLANTIC BOOKS
BERKELEY, CALIFORNIA

Chen Style Taijiquan: The Source of Taiji Boxing

Published by

North Atlantic Books
P.O. Box 12327
Berkeley, California 94712

Cover calligraphy by Chen Xiaowang
Cover and book design by Jennifer Dunn
Printed in the United States of America

Chen Style Taijiquan: The Source of Taiji Boxing is sponsored by the Society for the Study of Native Arts and Sciences, a nonprofit educational corporation whose goals are to develop an educational and crosscultural perspective linking various scientific, social, and artistic fields; to nurture a holistic view of arts, sciences, humanities, and healing; and to publish and distribute literature on the relationship of mind, body, and nature.

North Atlantic Books are available through most bookstores. To contact North Atlantic directly, call 800-337-2665 or visit our website at www.northatlanticbooks.com.

Substantial discounts on bulk quantities of North Atlantic books are available to corporations, professional associations, and other organizations. For details and discount information, contact the special sales department at North Atlantic Books.

Library of Congress Cataloging-in-Publication Data

Gaffney, David, 1963–
    Chen style taijiquan : the source of taiji boxing /by David Gaffney and Davidine Siaw-Voon Sim.
        p. cm.
    ISBN 1-55643-377-8 (alk. paper)
    I. Tai chi—China—Chenjiagou (Henan Cheng). I. Sime, Davidine Siaw-Voon, 1954– II. Title.

GV504 G34 2001
613.7'148—dc21

2001030942

02 03 04 05 06 07 08 09 10 / 9 8 7 6 5 4 3 2

Contents

Acknowledgements

This book has been two years in the making. The information has been drawn largely from Chinese texts, which needed to be translated, collated, and organized. We are indebted to our teachers for making material available to us, as well as for giving verbal advice and illuminating important points. Teacher Chen Xiaowang has kindly provided books and photographs, and also written the calligraphy for the book title. It was Teacher Chen Zhenglei who first planted the seed for the book, with his comments on the lack of Chen style books in the English language. His support has been invaluable. Our gratitude to Teacher Zhu Tiancai for his enthusiasm over our project, and for providing us with research material, photographs and calligraphy. Thanks also to Teacher Gou Kongjie for his constant encouragement and guidance since we met in China, and for writing the foreword for this book. In our quest for better Taiji, we have endeavored not to deviate from the traditional art. Along the way we have come across many teachers who have contributed to and enhanced our experience, for which we are grateful.

Above all, we acknowledge the love, support and belief of our families. A big thank you to Papa, Noel and Ita, Darren and Jehan. And *Xie Xie* to Ma, Chee, Mike and Ling. *Wo Ai Ni Men.*

Foreword

I have known Siaw-Voon and David for several years. In order to better their Taijiquan, they have travelled to China many times in recent years, in search of teachers. They have studied with Chen Xiaowang, Chen Zhenglei and other renowned Taijiquan exponents. Added to this are their own diligence, hard work and consistent practice, which have resulted in significant improvements in their skill. They have now decided to use their own realization, experience and understanding of Taijiquan, as well as knowledge gleaned from Chinese writings on the subject, to develop an English text to benefit all Taijiquan enthusiasts outside China. This is a very good thing and deserves commendation.

Chen style Taijiquan is a cultural treasure of China. It encompasses many philosophies that are applicable to daily life. Based on the theories of *Jingluo, Yin-Yang*, and the movement, self-defense and application principles of *Wushu*, Chen style Taijiquan has evolved into a unique and excellent form of martial art that is infinitely wondrous. Taijiquan enthusiasts need only study meticulously and endure the hardship of rigorous training to realize the benefits, be it for defending your body, for cultivation, or for keeping fit. The publication of this book is indeed good news for overseas practitioners, and for spreading and popularizing Chen style Taijiquan. Let all those who love the art join hands and toil together for the good of Taijiquan.

Gou Kongjie. Winter 2000

序　言

　　晓雯、大为，我认识几年了，他们二人几年来，为了学好陈式太极拳，多次来中国拜师学习。先后师呈陈小旺、陈正雷等我国著名太极拳名家。加之自己用心学习，刻苦锻炼，拳艺长进很大，现在把自己的体会、经验以及对拳的理解、中文版太极拳的认识，写翻成英文版提供给国外太极拳爱好者，这是非常好的一件事，值得庆贺。

　　陈式太极拳是中华民族文化宝贵遗产，它函于生活中的很多哲理，根据人体经络学说，阴阳学说，武术的攻防击技运动要求，形成奥妙无穷、独具一格的优秀拳种。只要爱好太极拳者细心研究，刻苦锻炼，对防身健体、养身都会有良好的效果。这本书出版对海外学者是一个福音，为广泛传播陈式太极拳将起很大的推动作用。让我们所有爱好者协起手来，为振兴太极事业而共同奋斗。

苟孔杰

2000 年冬

FIGURE I

The authors with Gou Kongjie at the Chen
Taijiquan Research Centre

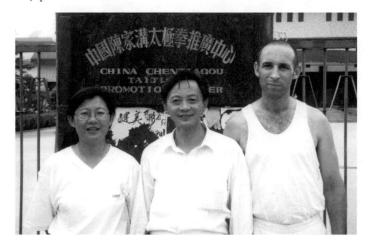

FIGURE 2
Verse by Chen Zhenglei

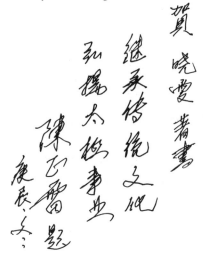

Translation of verse:

*"Bequeathed the Traditional Culture,
Proclaim the Vocation of Taiji"*

FIGURE 3
The authors with Chen Zhenglei at Chenjiagou

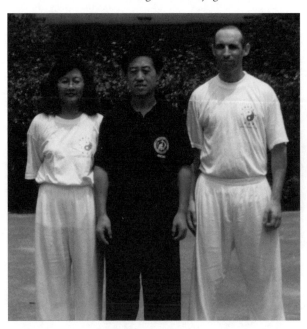

FIGURE 4
Calligraphy by Zhu Tiancai —
"Extolling Taijiquan"

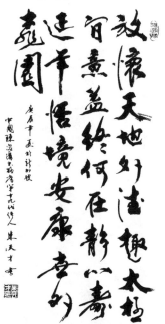

FIGURE 5
Zhu Tiancai

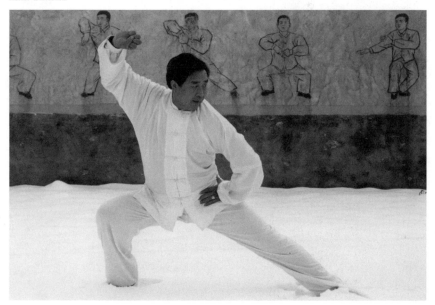

FIGURE 6
Calligraphy by Chen Xiaowang
"The Book and The Sword"

FIGURE 7
Chen Xiaowang

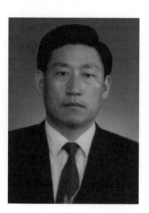

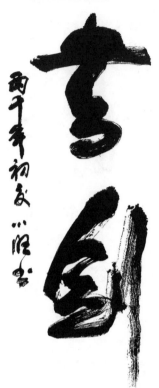

Chronological Table of China

Prehistoric/Legendary Period to 16th Century B.C.
Peking Man (500,000–210,000 B.C.)

> *Mythical sage-emperors:*
> Fu Xi-invented the Eight Trigrams
> Shen Nong—invented agriculture and herbal medicine
> Huang Di (Yellow Emperor)—invented writing
> and weapons

Shang c. 16th Century–11th Century B.C.

Zhou c. 1027–256 B.C.
Western Zhou (1027–771 B.C.);
Eastern Zhou (771–256 B.C.);
Spring & Autumn Period (771–476 B.C.);
Warring States (475–221 B.C.)

> *Birth of important philosophers:*
> Confucius (c. 551–c. 479 B.C.)
> Lao Zi (possibly mythical)
> Zhuang Zi (4th Century B.C.)
> Meng Zi (4th Century B.C.)
> *Yijing* (Book of Change)
> *Spring & Autumn Annals*—said to be composed
> by Confucius
> *Dao De Jing*—Daoist book (probably 4th Century B.C.)
> *Art of War*—by Sun Zi (c. 490 B.C.)

Qin (221–207 B.C.)
Qinshi Huangti (221–220 B.C.)—Construction of
Great Wall began

Western / Former Han (206 B.C.–A.D. 9)

Xin (9-23)

Eastern / Later Han (25–220)
First introduction of Buddhism
Silk Route developed

Three Kingdoms (220–265)
Pilgrimage to India in search of Buddhism

Northern & Southern Empires (265–589)
Buddhist influence in China
Military aristocracy dominant

Sui (590–618)
Reunification of China
Civil Service Examination established

Tang (618–906)
Emperor Taizong (military commander) (629–49)

Five Dynasties (906–960)
China divided into Later Liang; Later Tang; Later Jin;
Later Han; Later Zhou
First military use of gunpowder

Northern Song (960–1126)
Reunification of China

Southern Song (1126–1279)
Mongol conquest of China: Genghis Khan

Yuan (1279–1368)
Full conquest of China by Mongols
Marco Polo in China

Ming (1368–1644)

Emperor Hongwu, Zhu Yuanzhang (1368–98)—first
Ming emperor—ordered the "Three Cleansings
of Huaiqing"
Chen Bu relocated to Chenjiagou (1374)
Emperor Chengzu (1403–1424)—13-year search
for Zhang Sanfeng
Chen Wanting born (c.1600–1680)

Qing (1644–1911)

Manchus conquered China
Emperor Yongzheng—prohibited teaching of martial
arts (1727)
Emperor Qianlong (1736–95)—Literary Inquisition
(1550–1750)
Met with Lord Macartney (of George III)
Opium War (1840–42)
China opened to foreign trade and Christian missionaries
Emperor Guangxu (1871–1908)
Chen Xin began *Illustrated Explanations of Chen Family
Taijiquan*

Republic (1911–1949)

China returned to Han Chinese
Sun Yat-sen founded Guomingdang
Yuan Shikai-first president
Chen Yanxi *(sixteenth generation)* taught martial arts
in Yuan household
Warlord Era (1916–26)
Chen Fa-Ke taught Chen Family Taijiquan in Beijing
War with Japan and defeat of Japan (1937–45)
Civil War—Guomingdang v. Communist—
Communist victory (1949)

People's Republic of China (1949–)

> Mao Zedong—first chairman of Communist Party
> Great Leap Forward (1958)—leading to mass famine—
>   one of the worst-hit areas was Henan Province
> "Three Years of Natural Disaster" (1960–62)—
>   20 million people perished
> Cultural Revolution—destruction and banning of all
>   things traditional—martial arts practice prohibited
> Deng Xiaoping as leader (1978)—proclaimed
>   *"taijiquan is good"*

Note on Chinese names and terms

Chinese names are written in pinyin form, which is pronounced phonetically. Chief idiosyncrasies are:

Consonants
c is pronounced like **ts** (tsetse fly)
q is pronounced like **ch** (chin)
x is pronounced like **sh** (sheep)
zh is pronounced like **j** (jump)

Vowels
e is pronounced like an **er** with a silent r (tal<u>e</u>nt)
e before ng is pronounced like **u** (rung)
o is pronounced like **aw** (law)
ou is pronounced like **o** (go)

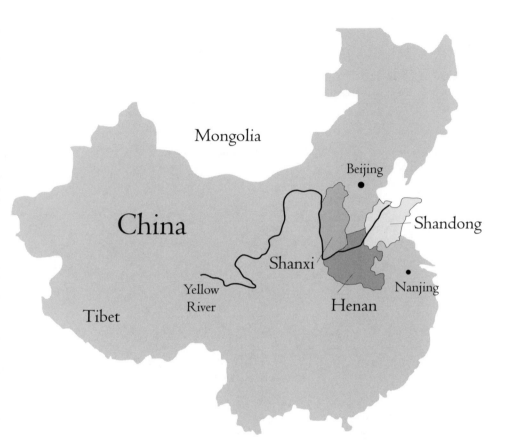

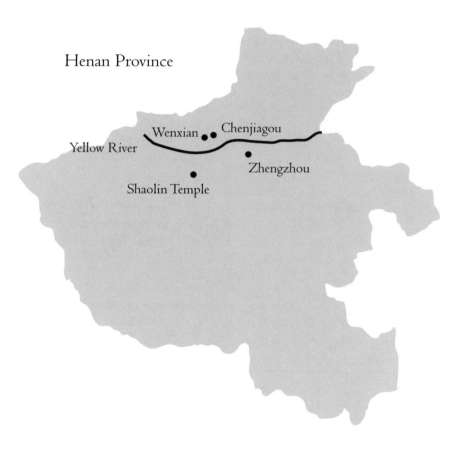

Introduction

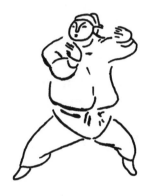

Considered for centuries to be a cultural treasure of China, Taijiquan has now become a gift to the entire world. Conservative estimates suggest that in China up to thirty million practitioners daily engage in Taijiquan, and media portrayals of this ancient and holistic art have proven irresistible in the West. When hearing the word *"Taiji,"* most Westerners immediately conjure up images of elderly Chinese practicing serenely in city parks. Touching upon the experience of hundreds of thousands of people directly, the oldest of the so-called soft or internal martial arts has provided the gateway for many to a deeper appreciation of Chinese philosophy, medicine and language.

That one might achieve optimum health, confidence and calmness through the practice of a powerful and effective combat system seems contradictory, to say the least. However, Chen family Taijiquan is underpinned by a philosophy curiously detached from the art of war. The embodiment of the term "martial art," the practices of Taijiquan is based upon a profound body of principles, theories and techniques.

Chen style Taijiquan was created by Chen Wangting, a seventeenth century royal guard from what is known today as Chenjiagou Village in Wenxian County, Henan Province. Shrouded in secrecy even in China until the early twentieth century, Chen Taijiquan is now practiced widely, not only in China and the Far East, but throughout the Western world.

The changing political climate at the end of the Ming Dynasty (1368–1644) and the beginning of the Qing Dynasty (1644–1911) led Chen Wangting, of the ninth generation of the Chen Clan, to retire to Chenjiagou Village. A garrison commander and government official, he was fiercely opposed to the new rule of the Qing Dynasty. With the fall of the incumbent Ming Dynasty, Chen Wangting's well-known support meant that his life was in serious danger from the new Qing rulers. Forced to flee, he eventually returned to his village, where he was hidden from the government authorities for many years by the local community. He spent the remainder of his life simply, farming, studying and teaching the martial arts.

Historically, Chen Taijiquan was developed as an eclectic fighting system incorporating many of the most effective techniques from the famous Ming General Qi Jiguang's *Canon of Boxing*. Qi Jiguang's system consisted of thirty-two martial techniques derived from sixteen major forms of Chinese boxing. Inspired by Qi's military text, Chen Wangting created five Taijiquan routines; a *Changquan* (Long Boxing) routine consisting of one hundred and eight forms; and a *Paocui* (Cannon Fist) routine.

Before the invention of firearms, the purpose and attitude of martial arts was serious, as the security of country, village, community, family and individual depended on it. Survival was its foremost purpose, not the health, meditative or aesthetic qualities, although practitioners did derive considerable health benefits as a by-product of the art. Successive generations of Chen family boxers earned their livelihood acting as escorts for rich merchants transporting valuables through the surrounding provinces. Faced with many challenges and dangers, their skills were developed to an extraordinarily high level. Many legends have been recorded of their exploits, which serve as an inspiration to the present generation.

Central to Chen Wangting's boxing method was the ancient

concept of *Yin* and *Yang*, the all-encompassing notion of complementary opposites that underpins Chinese culture and philosophy to the present day. Yin and yang represent the perpetual process of change and flux in nature, such as night and day, female and male, decay and growth, etc. Whether a thing is classified as yin or yang depends on the role it plays in relation to other things, and not on its own intrinsic nature. Chinese philosophy is based on the concept of harmonizing with nature rather than dominating it in an effort to make it conform to human desires (which is the Western philosophy of humanity as the center, with nature to be "conquered" to suit its sensibility). Humanity, therefore, is part of nature to the Chinese, and as such, this theory underpins all aspects of life.

Within the parameters of Taijiquan, the yin and yang theory is applied in a practical way. The aim is to harmonize opposing elements until they reach a state of balance. This will allow the optimum benefits to accrue, be they physical or mental, for health or for martial skill. For example, movements that are slow and relaxed are yin, and movements that are fast and strong are yang; closing movements where energy is being stored are yin, and opening movements where energy is being released are yang; the non-weight-bearing side of the body is considered yin, and the weight-bearing side of the body is yang; and so on. Taijiquan demands that there is no violation of the principle; that there is a constant interchange of yin and yang; that there is always some yin in yang and vice versa; and that a balance of yin and yang energies is always present. An understanding of the underpinning philosophy can help one to grasp the fundamental aspect of the art, as well as to bridge the cultural gap between East and West.

Perhaps the greatest innovation of Chen Wangting was the assimilation into his martial art system of the ancient health method of *daoyin* (leading and guiding energy) and *tu-na* (expelling and drawing energy), in addition to Daoist theories on consciousness guiding movement. This unique synthesis represents the origin of all Taijiquan styles. The combination of the coordinated movements of the hands, body, eyes and footwork of the martial arts with the techniques of *daoyin* and *tu-na* led to Taijiquan's evolution into a comprehensive system of exercises. Characterized by a joining of inner and outer power, the correct practice is said to require "training the breath inwardly, and the muscles, bones and skin outwardly." By incorporating the practice of *daoyin* and *tu-na* into the martial exercises, Taijiquan became a holistic training system in which the practitioners' mental concentration, breathing and movements are intimately co-ordinated. This paved the way for Taijiquan's future use as an exercise system suitable for all, regardless of age and health status, and applicable to all aspects of health care.

For five generations the skill remained a closely guarded secret taught only within the Chen family. Given that their very survival was dependant upon their fighting skills, the reluctance of the Chen family to share their knowledge with outsiders is understandable. Not until the time of Chen Changxing (1771–1853), the fourteenth-generation standard bearer of Chen Taijiquan, was the art taught to an outsider, Yang Luchan (1799–1872).

Yang Luchan went to Beijing after leaving Chenjiagou, where he modified the routine he had learned from his teacher, adapting it to suit people whose main goal in learning was to keep fit. This became known as Yang style Taijiquan. Omitted were many of the explosive movements, deep postures, stamping and variations in tempo that identify the Chen style. Over the course of the next two generations of the Yang family, the Yang style was further revised until Yang Chengfu, grandson of Yang Luchan, developed the "Big Frame" which has become the most widely practiced form of Taijiquan both in China and throughout the world. Characterized by slow, steady and flowing movements, this was the form that Yang Chengfu taught as he travelled throughout China.

While Yang Taijiquan and the other major styles were being propagated all over China, Chen style continued to be practiced almost exclusively in Chenjiagou. Despite being the source of Taijiquan "shadow boxing," it remained the least understood of the major styles. Chen style Taijiquan truly became a public art as late as 1928, when Chen Fa-ke (1887–1957) of the seventeenth generation of Chen Clan came to Beijing at the invitation of his nephew to teach the family art. His demonstrations caused astonishment among Taiji circles familiar only with the slow and gentle manifestation of Taijiquan. The use of swift movements, stamping of the feet, leaping and dodging, and explosive *fajing* (emitting energy) actions caused some observers to question how this could be Taijiquan.

Chen style Taijiquan is a powerful and effective Chinese internal martial art. Understanding of and competence in its fundamental principles are a prerequisite for anyone who wishes to achieve the greatest benefit from practice. Without a clear goal and understanding, a lifetime's practice may be futile. The foundation of Chen Taijiquan is built upon several centuries of accumulated wisdom and experience. Physical development needs to be accompanied by mental and character development. Knowledge and understanding of the requirements of Taijiquan can give insight into the depth and complexity of the art. Knowledge includes history, theory, philosophy and principles, as well as basic training requirements and methods. Although knowledge is no substitute for practical training, it can help one gain a clear idea of what is to be achieved and how technique must be manifested. Acquiring understanding is best achieved through practical training and direct experience. The important thing is to convert the breadth of knowledge into practical application.

All practice should be "according to the principles" (*an zhe gui ju*). The principles start with the basics and progress gradually to the highest levels. The key is to begin at the fundamental level and work step by step towards each level of skill. Taijiquan does not require that students begin with complex techniques. They must begin by understanding essential body requirements, performing basic body movements, and training to develop sufficient internal as well as external strength to execute these actions.

Chen Taijiquan has a comprehensive training system comprised of standing-pole exercise, single-movement exercises, bare-hand forms, push hands, weapons and supplementary equipment training. As with any other sport or martial art, it is important to start with the fundamentals. With time and diligent practice, the body is strengthened and one learns a new way of moving. Each of the different training methods should be considered within the context of a larger system. Each aspect of the training process, from the standing exercises to advanced push hands drills is inter-related and necessary. Viewed in its entirety, the training process is like a series of overlapping steps, each building on the foundation of the previous one.

Standing pole or *zhan zhuang* is the most fundamental exercise of Taijiquan. Holding the arms in front of the body in a rounded position, the practitioner stands and quietly observes the natural ebb and flow of the breath. This seemingly simple exercise improves postural alignment and balance, increases the strength of one's legs, and develops acute body awareness, deeper breathing and a tranquil mind. When laypeople talk of Taijiquan, they are usually referring to one of the barehand routines or forms, per-formed gracefully and slowly. The forms of Chen style Taijiquan, however, are made up of dynamically changing rhythms. Practitioners store energy slowly and then release it rapidly in a dramatic explosion of power. The style is often compared to thun-der clapping and then vanishing instantly; to a gentle breeze that becomes a storm; or to ocean waves crashing against the shore and then slowly retreating. Where the zhan zhuang can be said to pro-vide the letters of the Taiji alphabet, the forms allow one to write in complete sentences.

Push hands is a two-person training exercise created by Chen Wangting, the goal of which is to acquire sensitivity to the move-ment and intention of an opponent while concealing one's own intention and energy. In the "Song of the Canon of Boxing," Chen Wangting states that one should aspire to reach the level of "Nobody knows me, while I know everybody." Harmonizing with the movements of an opponent, the practitioner seeks to eliminate all tension and resistance within his own reactions. Unlike most external martial arts, the aim is not simply to block an incoming force with greater force, but to "listen" to and "borrow" the opponent's energy to defend oneself.

Taijiquan possesses not only unique external features, but also precise internal requirements. The focus is on *yi* (mind intention), and *qi* (internal energy) and not just on *li* (unharnessed strength). The first criterion is using the yi to move qi, which in turn moves the body's *jing* (trained power). In other words, in Taiji, one practices and trains energy by trying to focus and concentrate the energy from the entire body in the performance of each action. By using the mind, qi and the physical body, one achieves the three harmonies, as well as the ability to utilize whole-body power.

Qi is not a mysterious and magical thing. The ancient Chinese related qi to fire. In the modern era it is often likened to an electric current. Although not a tangible organic substance, qi is one's energy or life force. This energy circulates through the pathway of meridians *(jingluo)* throughout the body. Qi is produced in an area located between the kidneys and stored in the *dantian* (energy centre) in the lower abdomen. From here, it is distributed to the different parts of the body. Although qi continuously circulates within the body, most people are unaware of its presence (just as one does not feel the flow of blood and the lymphatic fluids). The sensation or awareness of qi usually begins as warmth in the palms or tingling in the fingers. It is also manifested as a feeling of fullness. The sensation of fullness is gradually felt throughout the body, as if one were expanding outwards in all directions. There is also the sensation of warmth throughout the body. Certain rules need to be followed to stimulate, intensify and ensure the adequate circulation of qi. Only when one has cultivated abundant qi will it be able to "push through" the gateways and "saturate" *(guan quang)* every part of the body, bringing with it the benefits of good health and providing the basis for martial proficiency. This requires consistent training over a period of time.

Today, although people seldom need martial skills for survival, Taijiquan remains an excellent art of self-defense. Also, considerable health benefits can be derived from it. It is a highly developed system of harmonizing the external body with internal energy. Its external movements stretch and strengthen the muscles, tendons and ligaments, while the unique spiralling and twining movements massage the body's internal organs as well as circulate qi energy throughout the body by the process of dredging the acupuncture channels (*jingluo and jingmai*). In China this important exercise is practiced daily by millions to preserve and enhance vitality.

Research by Western scientists has documented numerous health benefits enjoyed by people regularly engaging in Taijiquan. Health-related benefits include reduced blood pressure, increased bone density, improved functioning of the immune system, increased leg strength, and a lower incidence of falls among the elderly. In today's hectic and stress-filled world, full of competing demands and over-abundant choices, Taijiquan provides a means by which to quiet the mind and relax the body. Practicing Chen style Taijiquan encourages deep, regulated, natural breathing and a calm mind.

Chen Taijiquan is an inimitable example of Chinese martial culture, providing a tangible link to past generations of Taiji practitioners. Changed little through the passing generations, this art draws increasing numbers of practitioners by the aesthetic nature of its movements. It combines power, grace and agility, and is a means of self-expression for many.

CHAPTER ONE

Roots

Origin and Development

The birthplace of Taijiquan is Chenjiagou, in Wenxian (Wen County), in the Henan Province of China.

The story of Chen family style begins with the historical patriarch of the Chen family, **Chen Bu**, of Zezhou Prefecture (modern-day Jincheng) in Shanxi Province. He lived in the reign of the first emperor of the Ming dynasty (1368–1644). Chen Bu later moved to Hongdong County (Shanxi) and then immigrated to Huaiqing Prefecture (today Qinyang city) in Henan Province.

This was a time of war, devastation and chaos. At the fall of the previous dynasty, the Yuan (1271–1368), law and order were non-existent and the population lived in poverty and fear. There were frequent uprisings. The city of Huaiqing in those days governed eight counties, including Wen County. Its Yuan-dynasty garrison, under General Tien Moer, put up strong resistance, holding off Ming attacks and killing and injuring many soldiers. It was finally defeated by lack of supplies and reinforcements, and the few remaining Yuan soldiers dispersed.

Zhu Yuanzhang, the new Emperor Hongwu (1368–98), vented his anger on the people of Huaiqing, believing that they supported the last garrison. He decreed the "Three Cleansings" of Huaiqing, which led to the mass slaughter of the innocent population of the prefecture. This left an area of several thousand

9

square kilometers desolate, with no sign of life in thousands of villages. There were no crops, only knee-high weeds and decaying bodies. It was said that if a gold nugget were left on the street, there would be no one to pick it up.

According to historical records, it was at this time that a policy of mass migration and wasteland reclamation was carried out. A migration office was set up in Shanxi Province in Hongdong County, and local inhabitants were forced to move to now-sparsely populated areas devastated by the war (one of which was Huaiqing Prefecture). Among those forced to move was Chen Bu. It was in the seventh year of *Hongwu* (1374) that Chen Bu relocated to Huaiqing. Since the traditional starting point for all migrations was beneath a scholar tree (*huaishu*), the saying persists today: *"When you ask me from where I came, the answer is Shanxi Hongdong Big Scholar Tree."*

Chen Bu was an upright and honest man, skilled in martial arts. He helped many people along the way and protected them from danger. Upon arrival at the prefecture, Chen Bu saw a place in the southeastern section, with the Yellow River to the south, Taihang Mountains in the north, and a wide fertile flood plain, and decided this was a good place to settle down. A village was gradually established with hard work and enterprise. Since Chen Bu was by then recognized as the leader of the emigrants, it was decided that the village be called *Chen Bu Zhuang* (Chen Bu's village). Although Chen Bu later moved away, the village still carries this name and now is part of Wen County instead of Qinyang. A stoneroller used by Chen Bu is said to be the present stone cover for a well situated in the northeastern part of the village. Older local people are still able to remember stories of Chen Bu and his family.

Chen Bu Zhuang lies on low ground and is prone to flooding, prompting Chen Bu to find a higher place situated ten *li* (Chinese measurement=0.5km) to the east, called *Qing Feng Lin* (Green Wind Ridge). After surveying the land, he decided it was ideal. The place was named Chang Yang Village after the temple there. However, Chen Bu was told that the area was often visited by bandits who came from the nearby hills to rob and plunder. Local officials had done nothing to suppress them.

After Chen Bu settled in, he decided to rid the village of this threat. Gathering his family members as well as the strong and young of the village, he led an attack on the bandits' den. The bandits were no match for the superior skill of the Chen family, and the region was now peaceful.

Chen Bu's reputation spread and he established a martial arts school to teach his skill. The practice of martial arts continued through the Chen clan from generation to generation. The numbers of the Chen clan increased until the majority of the village inhabitants were named Chen.

Areas on both sides of the Yellow River were frequently flooded. Many failed attempts were made to deepen the river. Parallel drainage ditches, therefore, were created to help deal with floodwaters. These came to be associated with families. Chen Bu's family name gave Chang Yang Village its modern name of Chenjiagou, meaning "Chen Family Ditch." The name *gou*, which means drainage ditch, was attached to "Chen family" *(Chen Jia)*.

FIGURE I.I
Chenjiagou has changed little since the time of Chen Bu

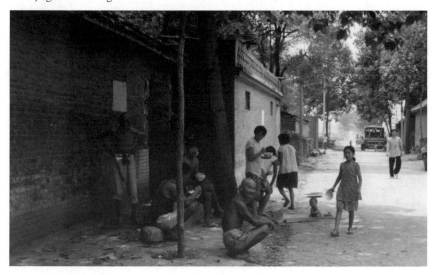

It is accepted that martial art was practiced in the village before Chen Wangting of the ninth generation, who compiled Taijiquan. It has been suggested that the martial art practiced was external in nature. The close proximity of the village to the Shaolin Temple gives credence to the theory that it may have been some form of Shaolin Boxing. The Chen family was famous for several generations for their *Paocui* (Cannon Fist) boxing and was known as the "Paocui Chen Family" *(Paocui Chen Jia)*. There were no historical records until the seventh generation, which revealed that Chen Bu had four grandsons. In 1711, tenth-generation Chen Geng erected a monument for Chen Bu, and a brief written record was made of the life of their distinguished ancestor. Detailed records of people, events and martial arts began with the ninth generation, Chen Wangting, the creator of Taijiquan.

The *Wen County Annals* and *The Genealogy of Chen Families* state that at the end of the Ming dynasty (1368–1644) Chen Wangting was already famous for his martial skills, "having once defeated more than 1000 bandits and was a born warrior, as can be proven by the sword he used in combat."

Chen Wangting (1600–1680), also known as Zouting, was a good martial artist as well as a scholar, practicing his martial skill by day and studying all aspects of Chinese literature by night. His father Chen Fumin was a *Zhengshilang* (a highly educated person holding an official position through imperial edict). Chen Wangting was well known in the Henan and Shandong areas for defeating many bandits and robbers during escort duties for merchant caravans. According to *Annals of Huaiqing Prefecture, Wen County Annals* and *Anping County Annals*, in 1641, before the fall of the Ming dynasty, Chen Wangting was a military officer and served as Commander in the Garrison Force of Wen County. With the fall of the Ming three years later, his advancement was ruined by the change of ruler and he retired to Chenjiagou, where he lived quietly. In the second half of a poem written not long before his death, Chen Wangting reflected:

Sighing for past years when I was strong and sharp. Sweeping away dangerous obstacles without fear! All the favors bestowed on me by the emperor are in vain. Now old and fragile, I am left only with the book of *Huang Ting* for company. In moments of listlessness I study martial arts. In times of activity I cultivate the land. In leisure I teach disciples and descendants so that they may be worthy members of society.

It was during this period, some twenty years after the fall of the Ming dynasty, during the early Qing dynasty (1654–1911), that Chen Wangting compiled a unique form of martial art called "The First Method," combining various disciplines and assimilating the essence of many martial skills existing at the time. Concepts encompassed by The First Method include the following:

• **Yin-Yang Theory**. This is the universal principle of complementary opposites that underpins Chinese culture and philosophy. The concept represents a dynamic balance, and Chen Wangting devised movements that follow this principle. Within a relaxed mind there must be concentration. Within a relaxed body there must be inner strength. In this philosophy the Chinese place yin (negative) before yang (positive), because the negative is the Mother of the positive. Therefore there must be stillness before activity, softness before firmness. In Taijiquan, yin and yang relate to movements such as opening and closing, and qualities such as firm and yielding, fast and slow, hard and soft, expanding and contracting, solid and empty, up and down, etc. In the legs, yin-yang is distinguished by weight distribution that has one leg "full" in support of the body while the other leg is "empty" and capable of instant direction change. The same principle applies to the upper and lower body. One must balance yin and yang; movements should not be too soft or too hard. If only one aspect is used, the form is incomplete. The knowledge, understanding and utilization of this concept can lead to the ability to execute the famous Taiji saying of "four ounces deflects a thousand pounds."

• **The Techniques of _Daoyin_ and _Tu-na_.** _Daoyin_ means "leading and guiding (energy)" and _tu-na_ means "expelling and drawing
(energy)." These two primary self-healing techniques consist of
mind-directed exertion of inner force and concentrated deep
breathing. They have been described in Daoist philosophical works
of the third and fourth centuries B.C. such as those of Lao Zi,
Zhuang Zi, Meng Zi and Qu Yuan, as well as the writings of Hua
Tuo, the great physician of the second century A.D. Chen Wangting combined martial arts movements with the techniques of
daoyin and _tu-na_, creating an art characterized by the intimate relation of internal and external motions: _"practicing breath inwardly; skin,
muscles and bones outwardly."_ Taijiquan, therefore, involves the close
integration of mental concentration, breathing and movement.

• **The _Jingluo_ Theory of Traditional Chinese Medicine.** _Jingluo_
is the term given _to_ the main and collateral channels that comprise
a network of passages through which the inner vital energy _qi_ flows
and along which acupuncture points _(jingmai)_ are situated. _Jingluo_
are distributed throughout the body, with the internal organs as
the source. If the vital energy in different parts of the _jingluo_ network is in harmony, a person enjoys good health.

Chen created twining, coiling and arcing movements that are
executed smoothly through the turning of the waist, each one inter-
connected. These movements correspond to the _jingluo_ and _jingmai._
The movements are alternately expanding and contracting, opening
and closing, firm and soft. Qi is directed throughout the body,
beginning in the pubic region, driven by the twisting of the waist
and spine through the kidney region, and passing through the _Ren
Mai_ (Conception Channel), the _Du Mai_ (Governing Channel), the
Dai Mai (Belt Channel)and the _Chung Mai_ (Thrusting Channel). Qi
energy is sent upward to the fingertips by the twisting motion of
the arms and wrists and downward to the toes by the movements of
the knees and ankles before returning to the pubic region.
Knowledge of this theory enables attacks on an opponent's internal
qi. Combining this medical theory with fighting arts, in addition to
the techniques of _daoyin_ and _tu-na_, produces a martial art that is

powerful both in attack and defense, and capable of an extremely explosive strength. Chen Wangting, therefore, not only incorporated the *jingluo* theory but also further developed it.

The "Canon of Boxing" of Qi Jiguang. A famous general and outstanding strategist in Chinese military history, Qi Jiguang (1528–1587) was acclaimed for successfully defending China against sea-borne invaders. His tactics involved feigning weakness and retreating before the enemy. After leading them far inland and lulling them into a false sense of superiority, Qi's forces overwhelmed the invaders in a sudden and decisive counterattack.

Between 1559 and 1561, General Qi compiled his classic text on strategy and martial arts, called *Ji Xiao Xin Shu (New Book of Effective Techniques)*. This comprehensive manual discusses both weapon and barehand combat in depth. The most widely quoted chapter is the "Quan Jing" (Canon of Boxing), which depicts an effective and powerful repertoire assimilating the arts of sixteen different martial systems of the time.

Chen assimilated the essential theories of Qi Jiguang and added the novel concepts of hiding firmness in softness and using different movements to overcome the unpredictable and changing moves of the opponent, thereby raising external fighting skills to a higher level. Power is generated from within, he said, with the use of "internal energy to become outward strength." This theory is embodied in Chen's "Song of the Canon of Boxing": "Actions are varied and executed in a way that is completely unpredictable to the opponent, and I rely on twining movements and numerous hand-touching actions." "Hand-touching" denotes the close contact of the arms to develop sensitivity to react quickly—*"nobody knows me, while I alone know everybody."* Development of this theory is of great significance in the history of Chinese martial arts.

• **Devising *Tuishou* (Push Hands) Training.** The push hands method created by Chen Wangting involves two people, hands in contact, practicing the movements of Taiji, alternately using the directions of body energy. It serves to develop the ability to discern an opponent's balance and intent by tactile sensation.

Traditionally, the Chinese martial techniques of *ti* (kicking), *da* (striking), *die* (tumbling), *shuai* (throwing) and *na* (grasping) had developed independently and were practiced in isolation. While a few might be combined, they each had distinct characteristics. Because martial training often causes serious injuries when practiced in earnest, these techniques had been reduced to a largely stylized and imaginary type of practice. Thus, some of the martial arts could not be raised to higher levels. Chen incorporated all these techniques into push hands practice and devised a method whereby the practical usage and value of movements and technique can be realized and improved in a controlled and safe situation.

• **Creation of the Basic Spear Practice Routine**. A basic exercise drill using long weapons or "sticking spears," this form of martial arts practice was institutionalised by Chen Wangting. In this method, two people with spears in contact use circular movements to train body movements, leg techniques, and offensive and defensive maneuvers. The method provides an effective way for practitioners to raise their skill.

It is at this point that **Jiang Fa** ought to be mentioned. Towards the end of the Ming dynasty, Chen Wangting participated in an imperial martial arts examination, impressing all with his great archery skill. During the examination, however, he killed somebody and had to flee the area. He joined the leader of a peasant uprising, Li Jiyu, (opposing the Qing invasion) for a period before returning to Chenjiagou to live in relative secrecy. The uprising was subsequently defeated and Li and his family executed. One of Li's top officers, Jiang Fa escaped, and went to Chenjiagou disguised as a servant. The ruse was kept up during his stay there, and he was called *Jiang Bashi* (a term for bonded servant). In private, however, Chen and Jiang were close friends and did everything together— exchanging martial skills, working the land, teaching students. Stories of the two still persist today: "Chen Wangting accepts Jiang Fa as his brother"; "The heroes from Yudai Mountains become friends"; "Master and disciple from Mumenzhai demand

FIGURE I.2
Chen Wangting (front)
with Jiang Fa

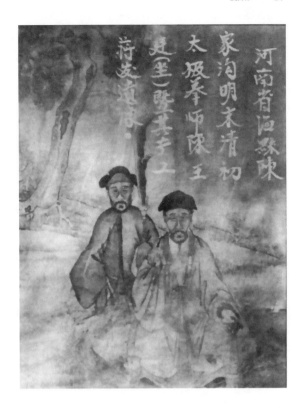

the cow." Jiang Fa was with Chen Wangting during the period of the creation of Taijiquan and made certain contributions. On the picture that is still kept in the Chen Family Shrine, Jiang Fa stands behind Chen, and his name was also recorded in Taijiquan boxing manuals.

The original Taijiquan created by Chen Wangting contained five sets of forms (one set of *Shishanshi* [13 postures], 2nd, 3rd, 4th and 5th routine sets); one set of *Changquan* (Long Fist) consisting of 108 forms; and one set of *Paocui* (Cannon Fist), making seven sets total. These also incorporated skills from the Shaolin Red Fist, Shaolin Staff, and "Buddha's Warrior Eighteen Grasping Techniques." Chen also added techniques from other well-known martial artists of the time, for example, Zhang Baling's striking *(da)*; Li Bantien's legwork *(ti)*; Eagle Claw Wang's grasping *(na)*; and Thousand-Fall Zhang's take-downs *(shuai & die)*.

Taijiquan emphasizes on whole-body relaxation, with the training of the mind taking precedence over muscles. The accumulated softness will progress to firmness, and change back to softness again, alternating and complementing each other. Quick movements are preceded and followed by slow movements. Slow actions should be slower than those of others, whereas fast movements should be faster than the fast ones of others. Chen Wangting, by absorbing the essence of the popular disciplines of his time, created a complex form of martial art. The earliest recorded Taiji poem is Chen Wangting's "Song of the Canon of Boxing," the use of every part of the body in combat, whichever part happens to be in contact with the opponent.

The Taijiquan skill was handed down and practiced by successive generations, producing exceptional martial artists in each. The Chen clan relied on their martial skills not only for survival but also for their livelihood as bodyguards and escorts. For five generations their skills remained a closely guarded secret, known only within the family and village.

Chen Changxing (1771–1853), also known as Yunting, of the fourteenth generation is credited with synthesizing the forms handed down by his ancestor. One of the factors that prompted this change was the high physical demands of the traditional routines. They contained many difficult stunts, such as jumping up into the air and coming down with a leg split or in a handstand; taking a crouch stance and circling one's head over the extended front foot; high floating scissors kick; and so on, making the routines unsuitable for even high-level martial artists when they reached advanced age. By the fourteenth generation, only the very skilled and committed in Chenjiagou could do the Long Boxing and the last three sets of the five-set Taiji Shadow Boxing.

From the five sets, Chen Changxing organized the main set of thirteen postures and the second and third sets into one routine of thirteen sections; he also combined the fourth and fifth faster sets with Cannon Fist (*Paocui*), making a routine that emphasizes powerful explosive moves, jumps, kicks and fist techniques. The two forms, *Yi Lu* (First Routine) and *Er Lu* (Second Routine), mutually complement each other and preserve many of the postures and all the movement principles of the original routines of Chen Wangting. This change from the original form represents the biggest change of all in the evolution of Taijiquan. The first routine is the oldest known Taiji form, from which all other forms of Taijiquan today have been derived.

Known as "Mr. Ancestral Tablet" because of his dignified attitude and upright posture, Chen Changxing also carried out escort duties to neighboring bandit lands, particularly Shandong Province. In addition to his synthesis of Taijiquan, Chen Changxing was the first to teach the secret family art to an outsider. **Yang Luchan (1799–1871)** of Yongnien, Hebei Province, went south to Chenjiagou to study with Chen Changxing. His diligence and perseverance impressed the master, who was persuaded to teach the family skill to a non-Chen person for the first time in their history. Yang Luchan was taught all the skills and techniques and later returned to his birthplace, where he spread the art. Many years

FIGURE I.3
Yang Luchan receiving Taijiquan transmission from Chen Changxing (statue at the house of Yang Luchan in Chenjiagou)

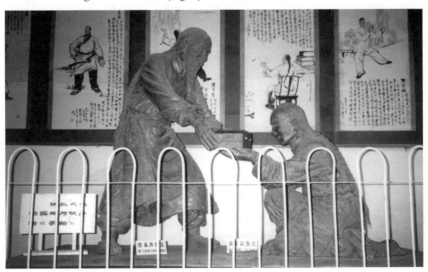

later, in his middle age, he was recommended to teach in Beijing in the Imperial Court. Here he earned the name Yang the Invincible for seeing off all challenges. In accordance with the condition that he would not teach the Chen family art to the public or use its name, Yang Luchan formulated his own style of shadow boxing. Yang style Taiji was based on Chen's first routine.

Also from the fourteenth generation, **Chen Youben** created another routine based on the original sets but dispensed with the more difficult movements, along with some of the more explosive ones. In order to differentiate the two routines, Chen Changxing's routine was named Old Frame (*Laojia*) and Chen Youben's, (*Xinjia*). The Latter was later called Small Frame (*Xiaojia*), as it is still known today.

The development of Chen family Taijiquan continued with fifteenth-generation **Chen Qingping (1795–1868)**, the nephew and pupil of Chen Youben. Further developing the form created by his teacher, he made the movements more compact, with many additional circles, in order to increase the realization of the application ability through practice of the form. This became known as the **Zhaobao Style**, as Chen Qingping lived, practiced and taught in the town of Zhaobao (2.5 km north of Chenjiagou) after his marriage.

Each generation of the Chen family produced very proficient martial artists. And yet there was a lack of written documentation of this superior art. The seven generations since Chen Wangting had largely relied on oral transmission. This was to change with **Chen Xin (1849–1929)**, a sixteenth-generation descendant of the Chen clan. Also called Pinsan, he was a grandson of famous Taijiquan master Chen Youheng, a brother of Chen Youben. Chen Xin learned the family art from early childhood and had very good understanding of its principles and methods. His skill, however, could not match that of his brother Chen Yao, as his father wished him to study literature. On seeing the martial achievement of his brother, Chen Xin decided to thoroughly research and make a written record of the Chen Family Taijiquan. His most famous book, *Illustrated Explanations of Chen Family Taijiquan*, took twelve years to write, from the 34th year of Emperor Guangxu to the eighth year of the Republic (1908–1919). Entirely written by hand, the four-volume book explains the principles and theories of Taijiquan, and the application of postures and guidelines for beginners. It put in writing the secrets of many generations of Chen clan Taijiquan practitioners.

The next major development in Chen Taijiquan happened in the seventeenth generation, with **Chen Fa-ke (1887–1957)**, the great-grandson of Chen Changxing. Chen Fa-ke was a sickly child and improved his health by practicing Taijiquan. He was not a particularly serious student until it became obvious that the hereditary title of "standard bearer" would pass from his father to a more deserving person. With strict family guidance and his own diligence, he became a recognized master when only seventeen years of age.

Chen Fa-ke is responsible for creating the *Xinjia* (New Frame), which is practiced widely in China and the West today. (Not to be confused with the routine created by Chen Youben.) Based on the

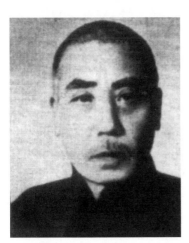

FIGURE I.4   Chen Fa-ke

Laojia (Old Frame), this also incorporates the *Yi Lu* and *Er Lu*. Chen Fa-ke made the form longer by adding nine more movements, for a total of 83 postures. *Xinjia* contains more complex *chan ssu jing* (spiralling movement), more *fajing* (explosive energy) potentials, more *qinna* (joint-locking) techniques and is more compact with more details. These changes aimed to enhance fighting skills and make the form more efficient in practical application, including combat situations. The same modification was applied to the *Er Lu* Cannon Fist. Chen Fa-ke lived and taught in Beijing for nearly three decades, taking Chen Taijiquan outside Chenjiagou so that more people could experience this orthodox style. His many students and now their students carry on their master's wisdom to spread Chen Taijiquan.

Of the eighteenth generation, Chen Zhaopei and Chen Zhaokui contributed in no small way to the promotion of Chen family Taijiquan. **Chen Zhaopei (1893–1972)** was also known by his pen name, Chen Jifu. He left Chenjiagou in 1914 and taught Taiji in different parts of China. It was he who invited Chen Fa-ke to Beijing in 1928. While in Nanjing, he published a book based on the earlier works of Chen Xin, and also created the Double Straight Sword Form. In 1958, Chen Zhaopei returned to Chenjiagou, concerned that the family Taijiquan was dying out in its birthplace. He is honored as the man who initiated a renaissance of Taijiquan in Chenjiagou and was responsible for the nurturing of such modern-day masters as **Chen Xiaowang, Chen Zhenglei, Wang Xian** and **Zhu Tiancai**, known as the *Si Jingang* (Four Buddha's Warrior Attendants) of Chen Taijiquan. Although persecuted during the Cultural Revolution for his teaching of a traditional art, Chen Zhaopei continued to instruct in secret. He even altered the traditional names of Taiji forms to communist slogans in order to be able to teach the art. His school and home became the inspiration and the location of the Chenjiagou Taiji Promotion Center.

Chen Zhaokui (1928–1981), the youngest son of Chen Fa-ke, joined his father in Beijing at the age of three and started learning the family art at the age of eight. He was noted as one of the first exponents of *Xinjia* while in Beijing with his father. He is credited for bringing this new form back to Chenjiagou in 1973, in order to teach it to the next generation.

Evolution of Other Major Styles

As mentioned, Yang Luchan, the first person to be taught Taijiquan outside the Chen clan, formulated his own **Yang style**

Taijiquan based on Chen's *Laojia Yi Lu* (Old Frame First Routine). He reduced explosive movements, stamping and jumping sequences, low postures and the tempo changes characteristic of Chen, while emphasizing more relaxation and softness. His aim was to develop hardness from softness. This modification was unfinished. Yang's version was adapted and revised by his sons. The second son, Yang Banhou (1837–1892), formulated what is known as Yang style Small Frame. The third son, Yang Jianhou (1839–1917), created the Middle Frame. The Small and Middle Frames were further modified by Yang Jianhou's third son, Yang Chengfu (1883–1936), into the Large Frame. With its slow tempo and graceful and gentle movements, this is the most widely practiced form of Taiji in China and in the West today.

These three generations of the Yang family were all excellent Taijiquan practitioners. They also spent considerable time and effort on the research and modification of Taijiquan. Yang style's Large Frame has the characteristics of being comfortable and extended. Movements are slow, relaxed and stable, executed in continuous flow. The forms in Small Frame are more compact, with quick, agile and light movements, with emphasis on martial applications.

Yang Luchan taught many students besides his own family. One of these students was Quanyou (1834–1902), a Manchurian who worked as a bodyguard in the Imperial Court. It was he who founded the **Wu style Taijiquan** (after the fall of the Manchu Qing dynasty, he adopted the Chinese name of Wu). His son Wu Jianquan (1870–1942) did much to popularize this style of Taijiquan, and is named after him **(Wu Jianquan style)**.

Wu style is a modification of Yang's Small Frame. It emphasizes the rotation of the waist, with a focus on mind consciousness rather than the circular movements of the hands. The feet are kept closer together than the Yang and Chen styles, and movements of the arms are also closer to the body. The form is very compact, performed in uniform slow tempo, and devoid of any leaps or jumps. A characteristic of Wu style is the back, which is kept slanted forward to form a straight line from the back foot through the lower spine *(Mingmen)* to the top of the head.

The three main lineages of Wu style are from Quanyou's disciples: his son Wu Jianquan to Wu Yinghwa and Ma Yuehliang (Wu's successor); Wang Maozhai to Yang Yuting then Wang Peisheng; and Chang Yunting. Wu style Taijiquan, with its emphasis on the maintenance of health rather than combat techniques, has many followers throughout the world.

The founder of **Wu (Hao) style Taijiquan** is Wu Yuxiang (1812–1880), a native of Yongnien, home of Yang Luchan. (The two Wu styles are sometimes confusing for non-Chinese-speaking people, as they have very similar pronunciation. The Chinese characters, however, are entirely different.) Wu Yuxiang was already a martial artist when he began learning Taijiquan from Yang Luchan, who had returned to his hometown from Chenjiagou. Wu was advised by Yang to seek further instruction from Chen Changxing. On the way to the Chen village, at the neighboring village of Zhaobao, he was told that Chen Changxing was very old and no longer teaching (he died the following year), and that a highly skilled Chen clan member was teaching in Zhaobao village. That person was Chen Qingping (see above). Wu studied with Chen for forty days, gaining a new perspective of the art. He later incorporated the teachings of both his mentors and formed his own style.

Wu Yuxiang did not teach widely and had only few students. His form was made famous largely by his nephew, Li I-yu (1832–1892), who is an early writer and recorder of Taijiquan principles and theories, and whose works are important references on the origin and history of Taijiquan. He left several hand-written manuals on the subject, and his song formulas and writings form the basis of today's "Taijiquan Classics." Li I-yu passed his art to Hao Weizheng (1849–1920), and it was he and his descendants who did the most to promote it and make it into one of the major styles of Taijiquan today. This style is therefore known variably as the Wu/Li/Hao style, after the three main exponents, and also as a way to differentiate it from the other Wu style.

The characteristics of Wu/Hao style are the compact movements and high stances. The body is held in a straight and relaxed position during waist turning and stepping, with each hand controlling its own side of the body and not crossing. The hands are not stretched out beyond the foot and toes. There is strict emphasis on rising, falling, opening and closing movements. Jumps and strength release have been removed from the forms that are practiced today.

The Evolution of Taijiquan

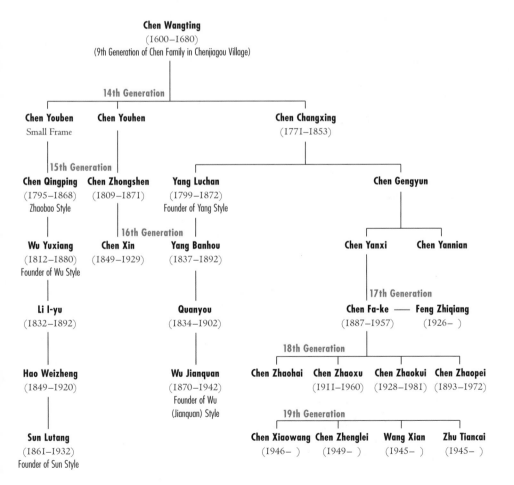

Sun style Taijiquan is the most recently developed of the five major styles. It was developed by Sun Lutang (1861–1932), a famous martial artist. Known also as Sun Fuquan, he was proficient in the two other internal martial arts, Bagua Zhang and Xingyi Quan. His form of Taijiquan incorporates key features of these two arts.

Sun learned Taijiquan from Hao Weizheng of the Wu/Hao style. Sun style, therefore, retains many of its characteristics like the high stances, even tempo, and minimal number of kicking and punching movements, but there is more emphasis on small, tight, agile stepping (from Bagua's footwork). Xingyi's leg and waist methods have also been incorporated. This style is frequently referred to as the "Active Step Small-Form Taiji." All movements are connected by opening and closing, so it is also referred to as "Open-Close Taijiquan." The style was passed on to his daughter Sun Jianyun, who continues his teachings. Sun Lutang also wrote several books on the three internal martial arts, which remain important references.

Recent Developments

Besides the five major styles, other popular forms have been formulated in recent years. Various exponents of Taijiquan have created these for different reasons—for general health promotion, for self-expression, for competition, for easier learning. Whatever the motivation behind the creation, the many forms have become widely practiced by no small number of people.

The most influential of the modern forms is the 37-posture condensed Yang form of **Zheng Manqing** (a disciple of Yang Chengfu). The form is most widely practiced in East Asia and the USA, where Zheng lived. It is one of the predominant forms practiced in the West, as it is quicker to learn than the Yang Long Form. Zheng Manqing's style is essentially Yang style and retains its theories and techniques. Zheng wrote extensively, and his works have almost all been translated into English; he therefore has a substantial influence on the Taiji communities.

The China National Forms developed by China's State Physical Culture and Sports Commission was a result of Chairman Mao's call for the nation to use sport to increase physical well-being. In 1956 a research team extracted 24 steps from the Yang style Taijiquan and rearranged these into the **24 Steps Simplified Taijiquan**. The process took six years. A longer form of 88 Steps, still from the Yang style, was later arranged. A further 48 Steps medium form was compiled which combined all five orthodox styles, but this has not been as successful, as the characteristics of the parent styles are lost in the mix.

With the inclusion of Wushu as an Olympic demonstration sport, the Chinese government devised one shortened routine for each of the major styles of Taijiquan. There are also forms that combine representative techniques of the various styles. These have gained popularity because of the official recognition by the Chinese government and the Olympic Council.

Chen style Taijiquan masters have also developed shorter routines to help promote their style. Feng Zhiqiang, a noted disciple of Chen Fa-ke, has done much to popularize Chen Taijiquan and created a short Chen form based on *Xinjia*. Chen Xiaowang created a short routine consisting of 38 movements, comprised of postures from both the *Laojia* and *Xinjia*. In recent years Chen Zhenglei developed a short 18-movement Chen Essence form from the *Laojia* as an introduction to Chen style Taijiquan.

The Question of Origin

The main branches of Taijiquan practiced today can all be traced back to Chenjiagou in the Wen County of Henan Province. Tang Hao (1897–1959), a martial arts master, undertook comprehensive research on the history of Taijiquan and concluded in the 1930s that Taijiquan originated with Chen Wangting. However, the origin of Taijiquan has been credited by many to Zhang Sanfeng, an itinerant Daoist priest of Mount Wudang. He is believed to have created the art after witnessing a fight between a snake and a crane. Many doubt his historical existence and view him as a literary construct. His years of birth and death are unknown, but according to different accounts he lived variably in the Ming dynasty (1368–1644), the Yuan dynasty (1279–1368) and even the Song dynasty (960–1279). His mysterious status was mentioned in historical documents such as the *Ming Shih* (official chronicles of the Ming dynasty) and the *Ningpo Chronicles*, which had no relation to martial arts. The earliest extant reference to Zhang as a master in martial arts appeared in 1670 in the *Epitaph for Wang Zhengnan*, composed by Huang Zongxi (1610–1695), when Chinese martial art was categorized into an "external" school of Shaolin originated by the Buddhist monk Damo, and an "internal" school initiated by Daoist immortal Zhang Sanfeng of Mount Wudang. Li I-yu (see above under Wu/Hao) in his *Brief Preface to Taijiquan* (1867) referred to Zhang as the originator of Taijiquan but rewrote the introduction in a later manuscript (1881) stating that the founder was unknown.

The legend of Zhang Sanfeng, therefore, evolved in three stages: prior to 1670, he was known simply as a Daoist immortal; after 1670 he was credited as the creator of the "internal" martial arts; and after 1900, as the founder of Taijiquan.

• The formative time of Zhang's life was during the Ming period (1368–1644), due to the close association of early Ming rulers with Daoism. Stories of Zhang Sanfeng's exploits and his magical power abound. The Emperor Chengzu (1403–1424) contributed greatly to the legend. In an elaborate ruse to locate the whereabouts of Emperor Jianwen, from whom he seized the reign in a coup, Chengzu initiated a thirteen-year search for the mythical Zhang Sanfeng. Neither was found, but Zhang was canonized in 1459. Throughout this period of the Zhang legend, there had been no mention of his association with martial arts, an omission considered very unusual in historical biographies.

• Huang Zongxi was a famous Chinese writer, philosopher and leader of the underground movement to overthrow the newly established Manchu dynasty. It is believed that Huang's *Epitaph* was a political statement against Qing rule. The external Shaolin School represented foreign Buddhism, which symbolized the Manchu rulers. The mythical Zhang Sanfeng, canonized by a Ming emperor, represented indigenous Daoism and provided an ideal counter-tenet to Shaolin boxing. A noted historian, Huang included a disclaimer as to the accuracy of the content of *Epitaph*. This piece of symbolic rather than factual writing, however, became the basis for the entry of Zhang Sanfeng as the originator of the "internal" martial arts.

• Emperor Yongzheng prohibited the teaching of martial arts in 1727. Later Emperor Qianlong (1736–1795) launched a literary inquisition that destroyed many writings from the period of 1550–1750 and kept writers censored for a further century beyond his reign. This could explain the lack of martial arts writings and references. Notably, this was also the period when a Ming patriot in a small village in Henan formulated Taijiquan. In Chinese culture, it was strict taboo to use the name of emperors (or in a family, the name of an ancestor). The name "Taijiquan" would not have been used due to Emperor Taizong (626–49). Evidence of this can be gleaned by the lack of any mention of Taijiquan in important documents such as the *Qing Unofficial Categorized Extracts* (1917), which contains a substantial volume of stories about martial arts masters and styles; and the *History of Chinese Physical Culture* (1919), which mentions 69 different martial styles.

• Xu Longhou, a student of Yang Jianhou (the son of Yang Luchan), established the Capital Physical Culture Research Association. In the *Illustrated Explanation of Shadow Boxing* (1921), he published the first known association of Zhang Sanfeng with Taijiquan. Tang Hao, who is responsible for the comprehensive research and dating of Taijiquan history and development, suggested that this was a conscious effort to arbitrarily impose the Zhang Sanfeng legend onto Taijiquan history, and saw this as an attempt to shift the origin of Taiji several centuries earlier to a celestial being. This book is the earliest available reference on Taijiquan, and those that followed, particularly Yang style books, tended to repeat the Zhang Sanfeng association.

• Tang Hao (1897–1959), also known as Tang Fansheng, was a famous martial arts historian who wrote many books and articles on martial arts and Chinese sports. He was considered a pioneer in this field. In the 1930s, he conducted extensive research into the historical roots of Taijiquan. After examining many Taiji classics, Chen Family manuals and chronicles, as well as other texts, Tang Hao concluded that Taijiquan was created by Chen Wangting of Chenjiagou Village in Henan Province, around the time when the Qing dynasty replaced the Ming dynasty. This finding is recorded in China's National Wushu Research Institute *(Kuo Jia Di Wei Wushu Yen Qiu Yuan)* and published in *The History of Chinese Wushu (Zhong Kuo Wushu Shi)*.

The origin debate continues. Whatever school of thought, one must not be too distracted by this. The most important thing for Taiji practitioners should be the search for the understanding of Taiji principles. Each style of Taiji has its own characteristics, yet in the structure of the form and the requirements of the body, they share the same principles. Over time the various forms may have changed, but the theory remains the same. All the masters of prevalent Taiji styles equally share the credit for preserving the art. They have devoted their lives to nurturing and developing Taiji through diligent and painstaking practice and research. Their methods are tested through time by the sole criterion of proficiency. Today, it is important for all Taiji practitioners to be open-minded in their approach and allow for open dialogue on all Taiji matters, not limiting oneself to the influence of a currently popular viewpoint.

Chapter Two

Philosophy and Theory

Taijiquan can be understood within the context of a constantly changing universe as a state of balance between the body and the natural world, as well as balance among the different components of the body itself. The need to attain balance throughout all aspects of life underpins Chinese philosophy. In the words of an early medical text, achieving good health is simply the result of "eliminating overfullness and making up deficiencies."

The Concept of Yin and Yang

The concept of Yin and Yang is perhaps the most fundamental theory in the Chinese worldview. Philosophically speaking, yin and yang represent the theory of duality. The idea is used as a means of understanding the nature and composition of everything in the universe, examined as pairs of interacting opposites. Yin is seen as a passive, negative state that is associated with femininity, cold, dark, quiet, night, and winter. Yang is considered an active, positive state, associated with masculinity, heat, light, vitality, day, and summer. Whether a thing is considered yin or yang depends on the role it plays in relation to other things, rather than on its inherent property. Therefore the relation of a yin-yang pair is not a static one, but is seen as a continuous cycle in which each tends to become dominant and receptive in turn. Night follows day; winter follows summer; the moon begins to wane when it reaches its fullness; and when a course of events reaches an optimum point, it will change into its opposite state. The idea of yin and yang was first introduced in the Yijing (I-Ching) or Book of Change more than three thousand years ago in China. Within the *Yijing* two symbols are used to describe the status of all objects being considered, an unbroken line "___" (representing yang) and a broken line "_ _"(representing yin).

There are a number of yin-yang Taiji symbols *(Taiji tu)* in Chinese philosophy. The most widely known version (Fig. 2.1) depicts two fish-like figures inside a circle. The black side repre-

FIGURE 2:1
Zhou's Yin-Yang

sents stillness or "greater yin," while the white side represents movement or "greater yang." Within each side is a small circle of the opposite color signifying the fact that yin and yang arise from each other. Also present is the idea of balance between the two forces and the certainty that extreme yang is converted to yin and vice versa. Named after Zhou Dunying, a Confucian philosopher of the Song dynasty (A.D. 960–1279), this symbol has come to be accepted as the traditional version.

FIGURE 2.2
Lai's Yin-Yang

However, in their efforts to symbolize and portray the relationship between the forces of yin and yang, Chinese philosophers developed numerous diagrams. The yin-yang symbol adopted by Chen Taijiquan as most representative of the art is that of *Lai* (Fig. 2.2). In this instance, the emergence of Taiji from *wuji* is clearly illustrated, as is the emphasis upon dynamic spiralling movement. Chinese philosophy understands *wuji* as the void or nothingness from which Taiji emerges and returns to. In *Lai's* Taiji diagram this is signified by the central circle within the symbol.

Yin and Yang Theory in Taijiquan Form and Application

Without a clear understanding of the Taiji principles, the practitioner can achieve little more than a superficial imitation of his or her teacher's skill. Indeed, the form may come to represent little more than gentle calisthenics and arm waving, achieving only a small fraction of the health and martial benefits possible from correct practice. Throughout the practice of Taijiquan the principles are multi-dimensional, frequently overlapping each other. This complexity is not surprising, as Taijiquan is an exercise whose goal is to closely integrate the internal aspects of the body and the external system of muscles, bones, ligaments, etc., using the mind as the cement that binds them together.

In addition to the varied combat techniques, *tu-na* breathing and *jingluo* theory, Chen Wangting also absorbed the Daoist notion of yin and yang. When applied to Taijiquan, yin and yang refer to hard and soft, substantial and insubstantial, fast and slow, opening and closing, ascending and descending, etc. In the words of the fourteenth-generation Standard Bearer of Chen Taijiquan, Chen Changxing:

> The ancients said: good at moving out and coming back,
> hardness and softness, moving forward and backward,
> [when opponent does] not move, like a mountain, difficult to
> know as yin and yang, limitless like heaven and earth,
> full and substantial like a granary, vast like four seas, dazzling
> like three lights, watching the coming force [to seek]
> opportunity, able to estimate advantages and disadvantages of
> the enemy, awaiting movement with stillness, handling stillness
> with movement, [all of the above are necessary, then one]
> can talk about [true] boxing method.

THE EVER-CHANGING SUBSTANTIAL AND INSUBSTANTIAL

In the process of training Chen Taijiquan, particular importance is placed upon substantial (yang) and insubstantial (yin). In practice substantial and insubstantial are present in the arms and legs, the left and right sides, and the upper and lower body. If the right side is full (substantial) then the left side will be empty (insubstantial). A similar relationship exists between the upper and lower posture. Coordination between the different aspects of substantial and insubstantial (left and right, upper and lower, etc.) allows the body to be balanced at all times, "comfortably supporting the eight directions."

The leg bearing the greater proportion of the body weight is said to be substantial, the other insubstantial. By clearly differentiating one's weight, the mistake of double-weighting can be avoided. "Double-weighting" does not refer to the weight being balanced equally between the two legs, but rather to placing oneself in a position that compromises mobility. Throughout the practice of Taijiquan one leg must be solid—carrying the body's weight—while the other is empty and free to move in any direction necessary. A clear understanding of this principle leads to effective rooting, allowing the practitioner to easily transfer weight during form practice or application.

Similarly, the dominant arm within a movement is substantial, the other insubstantial. The idea of complementary opposites can also be seen with the upper and lower body. While a rooted lower body gives strength, stability and solidity, the upper body must be relaxed, fluid and light.

One of the major goals in Taijiquan is the heightening of sensitivity to the movements of an opponent and the subsequent development of listening energy (*ting jing*). Listening energy involves sticking with an opponent and following his movements to understand the underlying intention. Once contact is established, the Taiji practitioner should gauge the smallest movement of the opponent. Chen Taijiquan theorist Chen Xin likens the hands to a balancing scale, such is the sensitivity required. The ability to distinguish between the two aspects of substantial and insubstantial enables one to distribute strength effectively during practice of the Taiji form, as well as to determine the balance of weight and strength in the opponent. To quote eighteenth-generation Chen family master Chen Zhaopei:

> If one cannot come to recognize how the weight moves
> distinctly back and forth between the two legs, then
> the upper and lower body cannot work together and connect.

If the upper and lower body cannot connect then you cannot absorb the opponent's force, you cannot use his force.

THE COORDINATION OF HARDNESS AND SOFTNESS

"Delicate like a virgin seeing a man, unbridled like a fierce tiger descending a mountain."

Within the Chen style Taijiquan routines there are numerous *fajing* (explosive release of force) movements, particularly in the second routine, the "Cannon Fist." This provides a dilemma for many people in the West who understand Taiji solely in terms of slow, gentle, meditative movement. While Taijiquan can be highly effective for improving health, fitness and quality of life, its training curriculum was developed around the eventual goal of martial proficiency.

Chen Taijiquan can be characterized by neither hardness nor softness. Instead it seeks to alternate hardness and softness until a middle path is reached. At this stage it can be said that the yin-yang principle has been realized. The essential path of training is relaxation *(song)* leading to softness *(rou)*. From the ensuing soft and relaxed state hardness *(gang)* develops. With the use of the silk-reeling energy, the softness can be highly concentrated, so that it is focused on one particular point. Through rapid emission it becomes hard. At the extreme of hardness, softness again follows, completing the cycle.

The practitioner alternates and coordinates the two forces so that, in practice, the form should be relaxed, soft and balanced, outwardly calm but inwardly strong, "like a needle hidden in cotton wool."

Taijiquan and Daoism

There exists an ancient tradition in China of movement and exercise systems associated with Daoism. Manuscripts depicting medical gymnastics were among the documents discovered in the Han dynasty tomb, dating from 168 B.C., excavated at Mawangdui. Among them were exercises imitating the stereotyped gestures of animals such as the tiger, bear, deer, monkey and owl. Devised to promote suppleness and relaxation and to improve circulation, these exercises contributed to the climate from which Taiji was born.

The Chinese word *Dao* can be translated simply as "The Way." In the context of the pure and philosophical form of Daoism, this is understood to be the way of nature. For its most important sacred text, Daoism refers back to the *Dao De Jing*, generally attributed to Lao Zi, a mythical sage from roughly the same period as Confucius (c.551–c.497 B.C.). An examination of Lao Zi's *Dao De Jing* reveals a number of interesting parallels with the movement philosophy of Taiji:

- Yield and overcome;
  Bend and be straight. *(Dao De Jing 22)*
- He who stands on tiptoe is not steady.
  He who strides cannot maintain the pace. *(Dao De Jing 24)*
- The heavy is the root of the light;
  The still is the master of unrest. *(Dao De Jing 26)*
- This is called perception of the nature of things.
  Soft and weak overcome hard and strong. *(Dao De Jing 36)*
- The ten thousand things carry yin and embrace yang.
  They achieve harmony by combining these forces. *(Dao De Jing 42)*
- The softest thing in the universe
  Overcomes the hardest thing in the universe. *(Dao De Jing 43)*
- What is firmly established cannot be uprooted,
  What is firmly grasped cannot slip away. *(Dao De Jing 54)*
- Therefore the stiff and unbending is the disciple of death.
  The gentle and yielding is the disciple of life. *(Dao De Jing 76)*
- Under heaven nothing is more soft and yielding than water,
  Yet for attacking the solid and strong, nothing is better.
  (Dao De Jing 78)

Softness overcoming hardness is one of the fundamental strategic principles of Taijiquan as a martial system. To the Daoist philosophers, water was a symbol for the characteristics of flowing and spreading. Following this theme, the concept of *Wu-wei* or non-action provides a central tenet of Daoism and has been incorporated in many Chinese texts on military strategy. *Wu-wei* refers not so much to inactivity as to remaining still when that is in harmony with the flow of events. One of the features that defines Taijiquan as an internal martial art is the search for stillness within movement, and movement within stillness. External arts are built upon a foundation of strength and movement. Taijiquan incorporates the extra dimensions of awareness and stillness. Though the body moves, the mind remains quiet.

Traditional Chinese philosophy emphasizes the harmonious association between man, nature and the universe. Taijiquan has assimilated this philosophic reasoning. Within Taijiquan practice, the effort to keep all one's energies complete is first and foremost a search for equilibrium.

Another sacred Daoist text is the book of parables of Zhuang Zi, which expresses Daoist notions allegorically. The writings of Zhuang Zi stress the importance of maintaining harmony and balance. For example:

> [The wise man] would not lean forward or backward to
> accommodate. This is called tranquillity on disturbance,
> that it is especially in the midst of disturbance that tranquillity
> becomes perfect.

The central philosophical underpinnings of Daoism and Taijiquan share the principles of softness, yielding, rootedness, balance, suppleness and maintaining the center. Within the Chen Taijiquan forms these influences of softness and minimum effort are revealed in the names of movements, such as:

- Plum Blossoms Scattered by the Wind
- Sleeves Dance Like Turning Flowers
- Cloud Hands

Likewise, the basic Daoist concern with the contemplation

and appreciation of nature represents the source of numerous Taiji movements, for instance:

- White Crane Spreads Its Wings
- High Pat on Horse
- Part the Wild Horse's Mane
- White Ape Presents Fruit
- Step Back and Mount the Tiger
- White Snake Spits Its Tongue
- Separate Grass to Seek Snake
- Ancient Tree Wraps Its Roots
- Eagle and Bear Battle with their Wits
- Swallow Pecks the Soil

In seeking to make sense of their own existence, Daoist sages observed and studied the celestial cycles. Earliest observations involved the apparent rotation of the sun and moon. The sun and earthly phenomena were examined during daylight hours, the moon and stars at night. Through studying the heavens they came to recognzse underlying laws and patterns of change. The characteristic circling movements of Taijiquan put the adept in harmony with the movement of the stars and the natural cycle of water as it rises in clouds and descends in rain.

Daoist cosmology postulates a state of primordial chaos at the beginning of Heaven and Earth. During this period the whole universe existed in a diffuse, undifferentiated and potential state. Following the action of cyclical time the energy of the universe divided and separated. Through prolonged observation, early Daoist adepts deduced that the light, transparent energy or qi rose to form Heaven, with the heavy, turbid qi sinking to form the Earth.

Chen Taijiquan theory closely reflects the Daoist ideas of separating the heavy and light qi. When practicing Taijiquan, the lower half of the body contains *zhou qi*, or opaque qi. The practitioner aims to sink this energy down in the body, making the lower body feel extremely heavy, stable and rooted to the earth. At the same time, the upper body is filled with clear qi, causing it to feel very light and buoyant.

Certain characteristics of Daoist astronomical and astrological studies have also been incorporated into the Taiji forms. These include:

- Holding the Moon
- Step Forward with Seven Stars
- Moon from Sea Bottom
- Pluck Stars and Change the Constellations
- Homage to the Sun

In Daoism great significance is placed upon not violating the laws of nature. Actions arising from partial understanding only result in imbalance. The book of Zhuang Zi states:

> The action of the sage is directed within. He does not seek to impose on the world rules, values, rites or laws that he himself has invented.

The only genuine law is that of nature, hence Daoism's attention to the natural sciences. For the Taijiquan adept, spontaneity arises from an understanding of the universal principles of nature. Taijiquan follows a characteristically Daoist approach, using the body naturally with dexterity and balance rather than resorting to brute force. Outwitting one's opponent rather than colliding head-on is the desirable outcome in Taijiquan.

Taijiquan in Relation to the Eight Trigrams and Five Elements

For at least three thousand years the *Yijing* has been used as a book of divination underpinning Chinese culture. The core ideology of the *Yijing* is the yin-yang theory and the *taiji* principle. As discussed above, the idea of yin and yang is also the foundation of the major Chinese philosophies. Within *taiji* are the dual polarities of yin and yang. The ancient Chinese understood the *taiji principle* as encompassing the whole or complete entity. The concept of *taiji*, it is said, can be applied to everything in the universe to allow one to view "the ten thousand things." Of central importance is the idea of wholeness. All actions and interactions are viewed in terms of constant and ever-changing progression, accompanied by an inevitable adjustment towards a state of balance.

"*Quan*" can be translated simply as "boxing." Taijiquan, therefore, was named to reflect the characteristics of an all-encompassing martial art. This wholeness is expressed in one of the fundamental principles of the art that states: Once moving, no part of the body must be unmoving. As Chen Fa-ke put it:

> Inside no movement—outside do not move—
> waist does not move—hands do not emit.

Self-defense ability is developed through strict adherence to a sophisticated system of movement, the body adjusting itself to be in a state of optimum balance at all times. Health benefits derive from the creation of a balance between the external physical aspects of the body and the internal visceral aspects. Chen Wangting emphasized simultaneously the importance not only of physical development, but also the character development of practitioners, so that a state of equilibrium could be reached between the heart, mind and body.

The *Yijing* is a complex philosophical system based upon mathematical principles. Within the *Yijing*, the Eight Trigrams are the building blocks of the sixty-four possible hexagrams (*gua*) used in analyzing variations in nature. Representing the eight elemental forces in nature, the trigrams symbolize the waxing and waning of yin and yang.

Together with the law of yin and yang, ancient Daoists analyzed and understood patterns of natural phenomena through the theory of the Five Elements (*Wuxing*). The five elements of Earth, Metal, Fire, Water and Wood were viewed as dynamic processes that could explain everything in the natural world. Each element possesses distinct characteristics ascribed after prolonged study of events within nature.

Central to the Five Element theory is the principle of mutual

FIGURE 2.3
The transformation of Taiji into Bagua (*source:* Chen Xin's 'Illustrated Explanations of Chen Family Boxing')

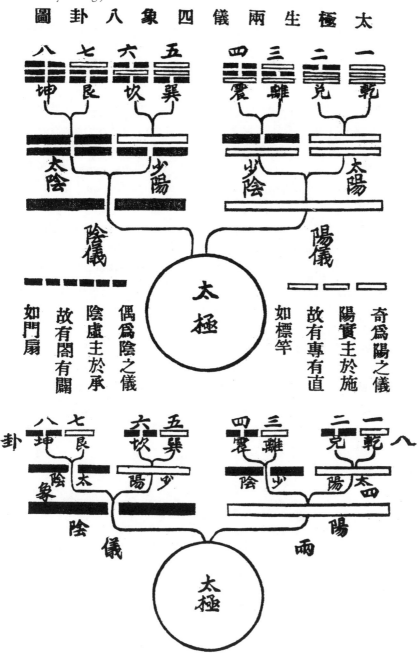

creation and destruction. Both creation and destruction occur in a cyclic and predictable pattern. Following the principle of mutual creation, Wood produces Fire; Fire produces Earth; Earth gives rise to Metal; Metal leads to Water; and Water produces Wood. (See diagram.) Within the destruction cycle Water defeats Fire; Fire conquers Metal; Metal defeats Wood; Wood defeats Earth; and Earth conquers Water.

An alternative name for Taijiquan is the *"Thirteen Postures" (Shi San Shi)* comprising the eight energies—*peng* (warding off), *lu* (diverting), *ji* (squeezing), *an* (pushing down), *cai* (plucking), *lie* (splitting), *zhou* (elbowing) and *kao* (bumping)—and the five steps—forward, backward, left, right and central equilibrium. The first eight represent the Taiji hand techniques *(shoufa)*, the last five its footwork skills *(bufa)*. Taijiquan theory matches the eight energies with the Daoist philosophical idea of the Eight Trigrams *(Bagua)*, while the Five Elements *(Wuxing)* concept is used to explain its stepping movements. The continual exchange of yin and yang that gives rise to the hand techniques and footwork of

FIGURE 2.4   Table of Eight Trigrams

Eight Methods	Trigram Name	Image	Direction	Associated Element
Peng	Kan		North	Water
Lu	Li		South	Fire
Ji	Zhen		East	Wood
An	Dui		West	Metal
Cai	Qian		Northwest	Metal
Lie	Kun		Southwest	Earth
Zhou	Gen		Northeast	Earth
Kao	Sun		Southeast	Wood

Taijiquan is also known as the "eight gates and five steps."

Each of the eight hand methods is equated to one of the Eight Trigrams and is divided into four primary and four diagonal directions. Eighteenth-generation Chen Zhaokui defines the relationship between the Eight Trigrams and eight energies in Figure 2.4.

The relationship between the five footwork skills and the Five Elements is shown in the diagram below:

FIGURE 2.5
The Five Elements
in relation to Taijiquan

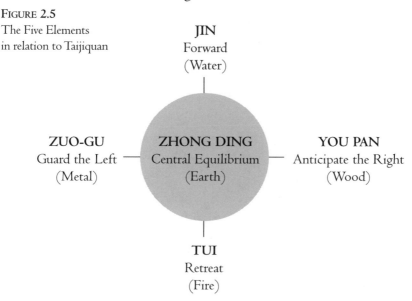

JIN
Forward
(Water)

ZUO-GU
Guard the Left
(Metal)

ZHONG DING
Central Equilibrium
(Earth)

YOU PAN
Anticipate the Right
(Wood)

TUI
Retreat
(Fire)

The central position or *zhong ding* is attributed to the Earth sign. During movement, qi sinks to the dantian. *Zhong ding* is a state of balance between substantial and insubstantial, allowing the practitioner to change weight or position at will. Advancing is given the characteristics of water, as one "seeps" into any weakness in an opponent's defense. Retreating is likened to fire. When stepping back, a strong spirit must be maintained to prevent an opponent from gaining control.

The Five Elements provide the foundation for the Eight Trigrams. The two concepts were originally separate philosophical systems until Daoist theorists incorporated them into one. In practical usage, footwork skills provide the foundation for hand skills to be effectively applied. Each of the weapons of Chen Taijiquan—sword, broadsword, spear, *guan dao*, etc.—is said to contain thirteen techniques. The number thirteen is arrived at by adding the five and the eight. Throughout the internal martial arts, this number is frequently used to establish a connection with Chinese philosophy.

Explanation of Qi

While Chen style Taijiquan is one of the most dynamic and useful Chinese internal martial arts, the attainment of its high-level skills comes not through concentration upon the development of physical strength, but through thoroughly understanding and utilizing the body's internal energy or qi. Qi is a concept that is as vital to Taiji practice as it is difficult to define.

The Chinese character for qi is usually translated into English as "vital energy" or "life force," although its literal meaning is "breath." No modern Western idea corresponds exactly to the range of meanings of qi. It is the central explanatory concept in the *Huangdi Neijing (The Yellow Emperor's Inner Book)*, the most comprehensive early medical document in China (c.50 B.C.). In an analysis of qi within the Chen tradition, nineteenth-generation Inheritor Chen Zhenglei suggests that:

> It does not refer to the oxygen breathed into the chest and
> the different kinds of strength *(Li)* in the human body, but
> refers to—from Traditional Chinese Medicine—Correct Qi
> *(Zhen Qi)*, Original Qi *(Yuan Qi)*, Meridian Qi *(Jingluo Zi Qi)*,
> Refined Qi *(Zhen Qi)*, and from the study of martial arts
> and qigong, Internal Jing *(Neijing)* and Internal Work *(Neigong)*.

Qi exists in the human body without form, color or substance. The ancient Chinese likened it to fire, and early Chinese pictographic characters depicted it as "sun" and "fire." Within Daoist literature qi was seen as a form of vital heat akin to sunlight, without which life could not exist. Today, the most widely used character for qi depicts steam rising from cooking rice. (The implication is that for water to boil and produce steam, there must be a fire, i.e., harmonization of opposites.) It is perhaps more easily understood in terms of an electric current.

Qi is formed in the kidneys and subsequently stored and driven from the dantian. A common misconception is that qi should remain in the dantian. While the dantian and *Qihai* (Sea of Qi) acupuncture point act as a focal point for qi, it is important to realize that all the body's qi is not collected there. Throughout the body, qi is present, with the dantian acting as a central co-ordinating point. According to traditional Chinese medicine, qi follows a pathway of meridians or jingluo. These pathways should be opened from the central dantian point.

Although qi within the human body has neither form nor color, its presence can be felt through sensations such as numbness or tingling on the surface of the skin, feelings of heat in various parts of the body, and a sensation of fullness like an inflated balloon. There is a great difference, however, between experiencing qi in isolated areas and consciously controlling qi through the various gateways of the body.

The development of qi comes from regular practice over a prolonged period. Inch by inch, depending upon the individual's aptitude and commitment, qi will gradually build up. Optimal qi circulation can be fostered through correct postural alignment, diet, breathing and mental calmness. The Chen Taiji forms, silk-reeling exercises and *zhan zhuang* (standing pole) represent the means by which qi is developed. Chen Xiaowang cautions that it is of primary importance that one does not try to force the movements. Only through being natural can the qi circulate appropriately. Practicing the form repeatedly, one gradually nurtures and refines qi. In the early stages the external movement of the body is used to stimulate internal energy. Once this has been achieved, the internal qi is used to drive the external movement. Internal strength (*jing*) can be understood as the acceleration of qi. Zhu

Tiancai, one of the "Four Buddha's Warriors" of the Chen Village, likens qi to a basketball filled with air:

> The air is like qi: static. It does not do anything on its own. If a skilled basketball player taps the ball and bounces it correctly, the ball can bounce up. Through acceleration and tapping the ball, the ball bounces up. That is Jing.

A clear understanding of the two fundamental forms of qi, pre-natal and post-natal, is necessary if one is to progress to the higher levels of Taijiquan. The qi acquired after birth from food, air and exercise is considered to be post-natal. As post-natal qi is not naturally present within the constitution, it is easily dissipated and lost. Pre-birth qi is the original energy that a newborn child inherits from its parents and is the energy cultivated subsequently during Taijiquan practice.

> If you use post-natal energy in combat, it is very slow and stiff. When you use pre-natal energy, you have a lot more energy for whatever you want to do. This original energy is the energy we talk about when we work at rooting physically.

> When rooting is strong and original energy is strong, then this person is very powerful and can work longer and more effectively.
>
> *(Chen Zhenglei)*

Silk-Reeling Essence of Taijiquan

One of the defining characteristics of Chen Taijiquan is its emphasis upon spiral movements. This motion is often compared to the central rotation of the silkworm's cocoon, as demonstrated when the silk is drawn smoothly, gently and without break from the cocoon during harvesting. Tai Chi classics recommend *"movement like pulling silk."* Reeling silk involves acquiring the thread in a

FIGURE 2.6
Illustration of Chan Ssu Jing
(*source:* Chen Xin's 'Illustrated
Explanations of Chen
Family Boxing')

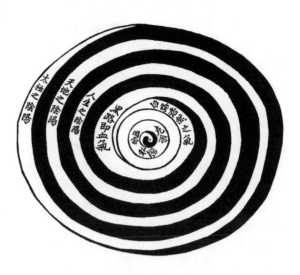

太 極 拳 纏 絲 精 圖

吾　極　打　明　絲　之　明　拳
讚　圓　太　太　纏　者　法　此
諸　圖　極　絲　絲　運　門　即
子　而　拳　精　精　中　也　不
太　悟　須　纏　纏　氣　不　明

spiral action, with the combined movement naturally forming a screwing motion. During training it is important to realize that within the screwing movement there is a straight line, much like the action of an electric drill.

To practice Chen Taijiquan one must fully grasp the silk-reeling essence. Silk-reeling provides the means by which Central Qi (*Zhong Qi*) is circulated around the body. Failure to understand this means that the system itself has not been understood. According to Chen Xin (1849–1929), "Taijiquan is spiral force … if you don't know spiral force, you don't know Taijiquan." The development of silk-reeling energy (*chan ssu jing*), therefore, is one of the fundamental methods of training Taijiquan and is necessary if the maximum health and martial benefits are to be realized.

Silk-reeling provides a means of eliminating stiffness and improving elasticity. All Taiji movement is achieved through silk-reeling energy containing the three components of relaxation, extension and turning or twisting. The omission of any one of these will greatly reduce the efficacy of the movement. An important goal of the silk-reeling exercises is to open and loosen the major joint areas of the body (neck, shoulders, elbows, wrists, chest, abdomen, waist, kua, hips, knees and ankles). At the same time the slow, even, twining nature of the movements stretches and strengthens the muscles and tendons, making them less susceptible to injury. Traditional Chinese Medicine views health in terms of the healthy flow of qi, which creates strong balanced energy to protect against illness. Blockage or stagnation of the qi in a particular channel leads to negative effects upon the corresponding organ and ultimately to illness within the whole body. In addition to improving the internal circulation of qi and blood, the *chan ssu jing* practice and the Taiji form provide efficient load-bearing exercise for the muscles and bones, leading to an increase in density and strength.

One facet of *chan ssu jing* is the even turning of the body. Even

FIGURE 2.7
Hand position during Chan Ssu Gong (*source:* Gu Liuxin & Shen Jiazheng)

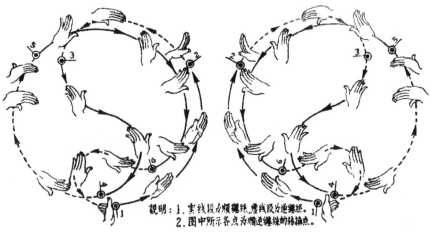

说明：1. 实线段为顺缠丝，虚线段为逆缠丝。
2. 图中所示各点为顺逆缠丝的转换点。

turning entails the adjustment of the hand so that it rotates to its limit at the same time the entire movement is being concluded. In simple terms, the hand and body must be rotating at all times. To turn the hand, the whole arm must be rotated. Similarly, to turn the foot, the calf and thigh must first rotate. Contained within the silk-reeling spiral movement is the requirement that movement of any part of the body leads to the whole body moving. There are no independent arm movements. In the case of the palm pushing outwards, the upper body is rotating the wrist and shoulder, while in the lower body the ankle and leg rotate. Throughout the *chan ssu* movement, the palm of the hand, whether it is from the inside pushing out or the outside pushing in, traces the shape of the Taiji symbol.

During exercise the rotation of the waist determines the extent to which the hands move and turn. At the instant in which the waist rotation stops, the hands should also stop. This requires the mind to be focused totally upon the movement. For generations practitioners have been instructed to use the mind *(yi)* rather than muscular strength *(li)* to lead their energy.

> Yi leading the qi, qi moving the body, qi swelling like a drum, and qi circulating in the whole body.

Silk-reeling energy practice seeks the unification of the entire body co-ordinated through the dantian. The internal energy originates from the dantian, with the waist as the axis sending qi to the left and right. It is distributed throughout the body by rotating the waist and spine. All energy that is transmitted to the extremities eventually returns and is stored in the dantian. This has been likened to the wringing out of a towel. However, this involves not just the hands but an integrated body movement with all parts acting together in harmony. The rotation of the dantian is central to Chen Taiji practice. While this rotation arises through the individual's movement during solo practice, in application it is a result of an external force. Training the *chan ssu jing* cultivates the feeling of rotation of the dantian.

Turning of the dantian can be visualized in terms of two planes of motion, or two movement principles. First, think of an imaginary axis running through the body from the center of the abdomen to the back. Using this as a central axis, the dantian then rotates like a wheel in either direction. Second, an imaginary axis runs through the body from the left to the right side. This time the dantian rotates in a forward and backward direction (see diagrams below). For the majority of movements within the Chen Taiji forms the rotation will involve a combination of the two axes. Silk-reeling energy exercises allow the practitioner to isolate the individual movements to clearly understand the underlying principle.

Teaching the practitioner to move in this manner until it becomes intuitive develops the martial application of the *chan ssu jing* exercises. Basically *chan ssu jing* can be divided into two aspects, *ni-chan* and *shun-chan*. *Shun-chan* represents the first half of the circular movement and acts as a means of neutralizing or redirecting an incoming force. This can be seen as the return of qi to the dantian following a path from the fingers, spiralling along the arm, traversing

FIGURE 2.9
Movement Principle Two

FIGURE 2.8
Movement Principle One

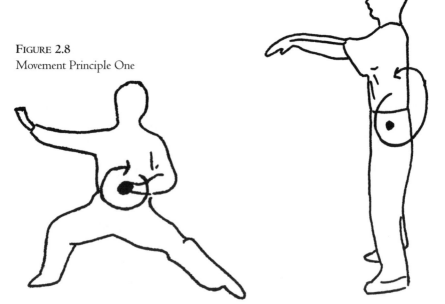

the elbow and rising to the shoulder before returning to the dant-ian. *Ni-chan* makes up the second half of the circle and, in terms of usage, is for countering an opponent using his own energy against him. The *ni-chan* represents energy emitted from the dant-ian and travelling out to the extremities. Again using the arm as an example, qi begins at the dantian, rises to the shoulder, and passes the elbow before being communicated to the fingers with the palm facing outwards.

The same principle applies to the legs, with *shun-chan* starting at the foot and spiralling back to the dantian, while *ni-chan* starts

FIGURE 2.10
Silk Reeling Path—Front View

FIGURE 2.11
Silk Reeling Path—Back View

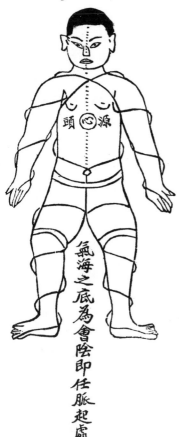

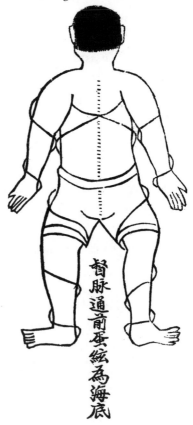

at the dantian and descends down to the feet. In terms of the eight energies of Taijiquan, *ni-chan* silk-reeling generally uses *peng jing*, and *shun-chan* uses *lu jing*. (See also Chapter Five.) These energies are present in all movements of the Taiji form.

Chen Xin's classic book, *Illustrated Explanation of Chen Family Taijiquan*, outlines three principal benefits of silk-reeling energy in relation to the martial application of the art. This energy can operate as a revolving energy similar to a tire rebounding any incoming force. The faster the opponent's energy comes in, the faster it is bounced away. This requires the body to be full, relaxed and sensitive. Second, silk-reeling energy can be piercing, like a spiralling bullet. This is a powerful and penetrating energy when applied during an attacking maneuver, whether it is with the fist, elbow or foot. Third, silk-reeling energy can act as a neutralizing energy, teaching the practitioner how to lead an incoming force to emptiness. Consistent practice of the forms with a correct understanding and use of *chan ssu jing* aids the Taiji practitioner in the development of *fajing* (energy release) and the eventual understanding of how to apply or counter *qinna*.

> In Taiji, the whole body is filled with winding and circular motion. Internal winding motion is co-operated with external winding motion. When one moves, all others move simultaneously. All qi power is delivered from the center of the mind through the inside of the bones, then transmitted from the muscles and ligaments to the tips of the limbs.
>
> *(Chen Xin)*

Chapter Three

Foundation

The foundation of Taijiquan lies within a set of principles that have been refined over many years from accumulated experience and studies. These principles are the fundamental requirements one needs to know and understand in order to be able to progress in the right direction towards the attainment of higher skills. The key is to begin at the beginning.

Body Requirements

The most basic principle relates to how the body should be used—*shenfa*. A correct posture is imperative for any benefit to accrue. An erroneous posture causes an imbalance and consequently blocks the flow of qi.

Chen style Taijiquan requires that one pay strict attention to each part of the body. All the requirements have practical implications for maintaining good health, for maximizing the efficiency of movements, for qi circulation, and for heightening the effectiveness of martial applications.

Head

In practicing Taijiquan, the head is held upright—*xu ling ding jing* (an insubstantial energy lifts the head). Imagine a light object resting on the top of the head, not heavy but always present. The neck is naturally relaxed and is kept flexible, as it must co-ordinate with the change in the position of the body. Do not focus so intensely that you tighten the muscles of the neck. The chin is pulled in gently. The acupuncture point *Baihui* at the top of the head is gently pulled upwards (Chen Xin uses the image of a string pulling the *Baihui* upwards). This, together with sinking down to the dantian and *Huiyin* points (between the legs), creates an elongating and extending effect. The alignment of the *Baihui* and *Huiyin* forms a center line around which the body rotates, and helps define the central equilibrium.

COMMON MISTAKES:

Declining the head—the habit of declining or dropping the head is often formed at the beginning when a student looks down to check postures and movements. The head should not bend down even if the hand movements are low.

Lifting the chin—this can be due to standing too erect and throwing the head too far back.

Wobbling the head—either vertically or horizontally.

Turning the head independently of body movement.

Eyes

The eyes are said to reflect the internal energy (*qi*), the intrinsic force (*jing*), the internal organs (*zang*), and the spirit (*shen*). In Taijiquan, therefore, the eyes should be alert and not dull, vague, or cast downwards. The eyelids are naturally relaxed, and the gaze is level. Chen Xin writes: "Eyes level gazing forward, shining into all four directions." This means that although the eyes are directed forward, one should be aware of one's surroundings. The spirit should be like that of a cat stalking a mouse. The direction of the eyes is in accordance with the body's movements. The eyes act as the forerunner of the mind: *"Of a hundred boxing skills, the eye is the vanguard."* It is the mind, not the eyes, which maintains inner awareness. The mind, via the eyes, gives the command. It is therefore important to keep the eyes and the intention of the mind consistent.

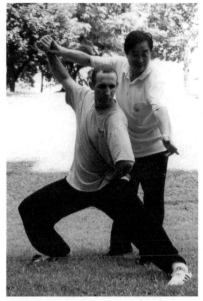

FIGURE 3.1
David Gaffney with Zhu Tiancai in 'Leaning with Back'

COMMON MISTAKES:

Unfocused eyes—the eyes are wandering and not focused on one's actions or intentions.

Dull eyes—if the sight is dull and lifeless, the mind is not in control.

Staring or tense eyes—a sign of tension or nervousness of the body and mind.

Closing the eyes—affects internal and external coordination.

Frowning—mind is not relaxed.

Ears / Nose / Mouth

When one is practicing, the ears are listening to an area just behind one's head. This helps maintain an upright posture, focuses the mind, and enables one to be aware of one's immediate surroundings (*er ting ba fang* or ears listening out to all eight directions).

Taijiquan requires normal, natural breathing; inhaling and exhaling are both through the nose. During *fajing* (expressing explosive energy), exhalation can be through the mouth. Breathing is slow and even, with the physical feeling of expansion and warmth. In general, inhalation represents the gathering of energy, and exhalation the releasing of energy, although this is not absolute. Breathing will be discussed later in this chapter.

Close the mouth gently and without tension. The lips are lightly touching. Keep the tip of the tongue resting softly on the top palate behind the front teeth *(she ding shang er)*. If saliva accumulates, do not spit it out, but ingest slowly with several swallows. Visualize swallowing the accumulated essence into the dantian. According to Daoism, saliva is the body's "longevity fluid." The saliva also keeps the oral cavity moist to prevent dryness, which can affect mind harmony. Another consideration is the fact that the yang meridian ends at the upper palate, and the yin meridian starts at the lower palate. The tongue acts as a bridge to complete the circulation.

COMMON MISTAKES:

Opened mouth

Protruding tongue

Pursed lips

—these are all signs of mental tension.

Shoulders

The shoulders are level, lowered and relaxed, carried without any tension. The relaxed shoulder *(song jien)* is achieved only through a period of focused training. One must not raise or depress the shoulders. If the shoulders are raised, qi floats to the upper body and causes a loss of energy in the whole body, as well as instability in the roots. If the shoulders are depressed, the internal power cannot reach the hands. It is important to avoid lifting, shrugging and, in movement, uneven shoulder level. The shoulders move as a result of changes in the body, and in accordance with the opening and closing movements of the chest. When the shoulders are raised, breathing becomes shallow and thoracic.

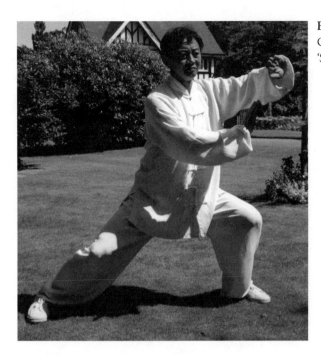

FIGURE 3.2
Gou Konjie in posture
'Small Catch and Hit'

COMMON MISTAKES:

Lifting the shoulders—this is a major problem. It lifts the qi energy upwards, thereby affecting balance and rooting.

Excessive shoulder movements—this occurs when movements are not manipulated by the waist. Often this occurs when a practitioner uses the shoulders to lead movements. Once ingrained, the habit is difficult to correct.

Huddling the shoulders—this mistake is often a result of trying to hollow the chest too much. The shoulders are rolled forward unnaturally.

Arms and Elbows

The arms are always rounded, forming an arc, with *peng* (warding off) energy intact. There are no straight or angled positions. When both arms are extended (as in Single Whip or White Crane

Spreads Its Wings), they maintain the same circular arc. The arms are relaxed and not pressed close to the body. There should be a slight feeling of opening. The space under each arm is roughly that of a clenched fist. This enables easier execution of deflection and neutralizing techniques.

The elbows are always kept slightly lower than the shoulders and are slightly bent and drawn in *(cui zhou)*. Drawing in the elbows facilitates relaxing the shoulders. When extending the arms, the elbows should not be straightened so much that they lose their function of protecting the vital areas of the ribs. When drawing in the arms, the elbows should not press too closely against the sides: *"Zhou pu li lei; lei pu tieh zhou"* (Elbows do not leave the ribs; ribs do not stick to elbows). Elbows can only be lifted when executing an elbow strike.

COMMON MISTAKES:

Lifting the elbows—a major fault that affects qi flow and also puts one in a vulnerable posture during push hands and martial usage. Elbows are always drawn towards the knees.

Wrists and Fingers

"Yang zhi zuo wan" means extend the fingers and seat the wrists. The wrist joints are opened up so that energy can connect to the fingers. The fingers are loosely extended and the wrists slightly dropped ("sitting"). If the wrists are not sitting, the shoulders, elbows and hands will be lifted. Flexibility of the wrist joints should not be overlooked, as the teaching explains: *"Chuan guan zhai chien; zhe tieh zhai wan."* (Turning depends on the shoulders, folding depends on the wrists.)

Extending the fingers means gently opening the joints of the fingers. Maintain a slight stretch in the middle fingers at all times, while relaxing the rest of the fingers. The thumb and the little finger are slightly drawn towards each other. This allows the palm to remain slightly cupped, keeping the *Laogong* acupuncture point (middle of palm) insubstantial. Qi is contained and the palms will not be stiffly held. The *Hukou* (Tiger's Mouth), located between the thumb and index finger, is kept rounded.

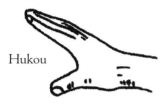

FIGURE 3.3

Hukou

At the end of movements, qi should be felt in the middle finger. Chen Xin: " *When qi arrives in the middle finger, it should arrive in all the fingers.*" When holding a fist, the thumb covers the middle joint of the middle finger. *Laogong* remains insubstantial but without dispersing the fist. In motion the fist is relaxed, tightening only at the moment of contact. Therefore the wrist should not be weak at the point of *fajing*, but full of *peng* energy.

The most common hand positions in Chen style are the open palm, the fist and the hook.

COMMON MISTAKES:

Curling up the fingers—lifeless and weak; energy will not reach fingertips.

Extending the wrists and fingers too rigidly—energy blocked.

Trembling hands—sign of nervousness.

Chest

The classic rule of Taijiquan is *Han Xiong*. *Han* means "to contain." *Xiong* means "chest." The chest is slightly drawn in, storing energy within. This allows the area to relax, eliminates tension in the ribs and allows smooth, natural breathing. The arms are free to move within a posture. However, one must not draw the chest in too much. The concept of containing the chest has been widely misinterpreted, resulting in many practitioners hunching their backs to achieve the effect. Chen Xin writes: "Chest stores energy *(han jing)*, but must also be insubstantial *(xu)*." Also: "chest must be relaxed *(song)*, so that the whole body is comfortable." Relaxation of the chest enables the shoulders to relax, which in turn helps the energy created by the legs to pass through the back to the shoulders and then to the hands.

COMMON MISTAKES:

Tightness in the chest—this may be due to insufficient fangsong (letting loose). Qi has not descended into the dantian and is accumulated in the upper body. Breathing may not be natural or co-ordinated with movement requirements.

Sticking out the chest—over-emphasizing the opening movement of the chest. When opening one should open the chest muscles sideways rather than forward. Lifting the chest creates tension in the diaphragm and affects deeper breathing. In combat, a raised chest exposes the area to attack.

Overly concave chest—exaggerating the closing movement of the chest. A concave posture places pressure on the heart.

Back/Spine

The back plays an important role in Taijiquan. It is held naturally straight and centered *(zhong zheng)*, and not arched or hunched. The area of the back between the two arms extends towards the hands for a rounded feeling (with the impression of both shoulders and both elbows very slightly "peng" forward). Chen style writings do not mention "pulling the back" *(ba bei)*, as this may lead to an over-arching of the back. The slightly elongated feeling is achieved by the correct posture of the head, letting qi sink down to the dantian as the feet grip the ground. Chen Zhaopei believed that pulling the back makes the body top-heavy, which affects rooting. (Chen Zhaopei is the famous eighteenth-generation master who revived and elevated the standard of Taijiquan in Chenjiagou in the 1960s).

The mainstay of Taiji movements and posture is the spine, as it links the head, the body and the limbs, facilitating whole-body movement. The spine is made up of the vertebrae. By keeping the spine straight, relaxed and strong, the gaps between the vertebrae will be opened naturally so that qi can pass through, up or down, very smoothly, facilitating ease of action. The spine should be like a flexible rope and not a stiff pole. If the spine is stiff, energy and power will not be transmitted from the feet to the hands. However, the spine should not be weak either, or the vertical wave power of the body will be limited, making Taiji force small.

COMMON MISTAKES:

Hunching the back—this commonly occurs when attempting to close or hollow the chest.

Collapsing the spine—occurs when the spine is weak and lifeless; this can happen when relaxation and looseness are misconstrued.

Waist

In Chinese terminology, the waist (*yao*) refers to the entire lumbar area between the hip bones and the ribs. It encompasses the lower back and kidney area, as well as the dantian below and behind the navel.

The waist acts as the central link connecting the upper and lower body. It is the "dominator" that controls circular movements, bending and the wave-like movements of Chen Taijiquan. Whether one turns vertically or horizontally, the waist is the most important axis. It is this area that controls the change of direction, and it is also the center of internal energy. It regulates posture, coordinates movements and maintains balance. The waist's flexibility, strength and agility are directly related to the body's ability to balance. Silk-reeling turning of the waist facilitates the building up of strength in this area. Fast twisting at the waist exerts powerful energy (*fajing*).

Below the waist to the front is the location of the dantian (three fingers below the navel). Dantian rotation is the essence of Chen style Taijiquan. Below the waist to the back is the location of the *Mingmen* acupuncture point. The *Mingmen* area should always be kept slightly expanded. Most of the power is directed through this acupuncture point. Turning of the body is achieved by relaxing the waist. If the area is stiff, the action of turning the waist may harm the spine.

Chen Taijiquan emphasizes *qi chen dantian*—sinking energy to the lower abdomen. Turn the tailbone *(wei gu)* downwards and the *Changqiang* acupuncture point outwards. Sit on the pelvic girdle as if perching on a stool. Relax the lower back muscles so that it can have maximum rotation. There is a feeling of pulling in opposite directions, 40% pulling upwards and 60% pulling downwards.

COMMON MISTAKES:

Not keeping the waist straight—this tends to be common in beginners when there is insufficient strength in the lower body.

A stiff waist—lack of movement in the waist prevents this part of the body from leading movements.

Excessive movement of the waist—the waist is too loose and moves and twists too much. The waist should be relaxed but strong, moving according to the Taiji principles.

Tailbone, Buttocks, Kua and Dang

The **tailbone** is naturally relaxed and *zhong zhen*—centered and correct. Its direction corresponds with the driving movement of the waist. In natural breathing, inhalation slightly tilts the tailbone inwards and upwards, aiding energy flow from the *Huiyin* to *Mingmen*, which then naturally rises to the *Du* channel. In exhalation there should be a downward relaxed feeling, aiding qi in moving down to the dantian and out to the *Ren* channel.

The **buttocks** follow the direction of the spine and remain perpendicular to the ground. Avoid protruding the buttocks or tucking them in too much. Incorrect position disturbs proper alignment, creates tension and prevents the legs from moving freely. Fixing the buttocks in one position prevents the smooth turning of the waist, which is essential in Chen Taiji's spiral and circular movements.

Kua is the muscle on both sides at the inguinal crease at the top of the legs. *Song kua*—relaxing the *kua*—is a term frequently mentioned in Taijiquan practice. The *kua* facilitate co-ordinated upper and lower body movements.

Through the relaxed *kua*, together with the spiral turning of the waist, weight change in the lower body is smooth. The upper body is then able to realize lightness or solidity.

Turning of the waist from left to right and the shifting of weight in the legs rely on the *kua* being relaxed and loose. However, the concept of *song kua* is not easy to realize. When the *kua* are relaxed, the weight burden on the legs increases. If the legs are not strong enough, as is common with beginners, it is easy to tighten up the *kua*, resulting in the knees extending over the toes, abdomen and chest sticking out, and the body leaning backward. This can cause injury to the knee joints, as well as a mis-aligned posture.

Dang (the crotch) should be held open and rounded to ensure agile footwork and smooth shifting of weight. It should be held in an upside-down U shape, and not an angular V shape. This is the area where the *Huiyin* point is situated, where the *Du* and *Ren* channels begin. The point should be kept light and without tension, in order to create balance.

Kua and *dang* work closely together. To round the *dang*, the *kua* need to be relaxed and open; the muscles on the inner thigh have the feeling of slightly pushing back and out. During movement, there is a close relationship between the waist and *dang*, and between the *dang*, the *kua* and the knees. The waist is relaxed and sunk down, *kua* are opened, and knees are drawn in—leading to a naturally open and rounded *dang*.

FIGURE 3.4
The dang is rounded at all times.

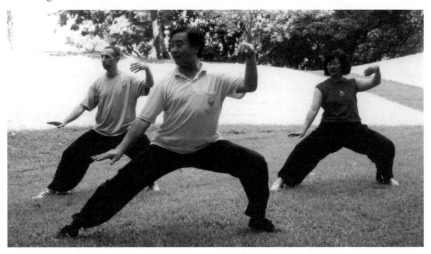

When shifting weight (i.e., interchange of substantial and insubstantial), the *kua* and *dang* move in a figure-eight pattern, made possible by the sinking and turning of the buttocks. The underpinning spiral actions of Chen Taijiquan make the movement smooth and prevent any erratic movement or protrusion of the buttocks. Move *dang* in a shallow concave curve (like a shallow wok) to ensure that weight is properly shifted from one foot to the other and that *jing* moves to the hands. This requires diligent practice to accomplish. The benefit of shifting weight in this manner is that *jing* will not be lost in between movements and will be delivered to the hands in a spiral.

Chen style's requirement of the rounded *dang* is strict. It should also be light, relaxed and flexible. Avoid the angular, rigid and collapsed *dang*. Collapsed *dang* is when the buttocks drop below the level of the knees. This locks the knee joints, making weight change awkward and footwork clumsy. The angle of the bent leg should not be less than 90 degrees. The *dang* area plays an important role both in the form movement and in usage. Keeping the *dang* rounded and opened increases strength in the legs.

Common mistakes:

Sticking out the buttocks—a sign of insufficient strength in the waist and legs to support the upper body.

Pushing the kua forward—this is considered a major problem. The top of the thigh is kept too rigid or too straight, is unable to sink down, and therefore prevents the waist from moving freely.

Collapsing the dang—when the dang is allowed to drop below the level of stability, i.e., below the level of the knees.

Not opening the dang sufficiently—resulting in an angular rather than a rounded dang.

Opening the dang too much—while opening the dang, the knees and the feet should be kept slightly drawn in, thus containing the energy and maintaining balance.

Legs

When standing, the inside leg pushes slightly back and out, while the front of the legs has the feeling of closing. This gives a sense of containment, as well as an opposing open-close energy.

The position of the legs determines the stability and balance of the body, as well as the flexibility of the upper limbs. The joints of the legs should be positioned correctly, so that power can be effectively transmitted through them from the feet. The height of a stance should be adjusted in accordance with a person's age and level of fitness.

Knees

The knees are kept slightly bent throughout Taiji practice. Balance is maintained by the alignment of the knees in relation to the hips and ankles. The knees are for movements and connections, not for support. Care must be taken not to put undue pressure on the knee ligaments and knee joints. When the knees go forward in bending, they cannot extend beyond the toes. The knees do not bend independently, but in response to the *kua* relaxing, hips sitting and the tailbone extending. The weight of the body should be directed through the knees into the feet (ground). *Zhan zhuang* (standing pole) can increase the strength in the legs. Proper warm-up of the joints before practice helps prevent injury.

When taking a step with *shun-chan* (flow), the knees open outwards. In fixed position the knees are slightly drawn in. In *ni-chan* (reverse flow) stepping out as well as fixed position, the knees are both drawn in. When lifting the knee (in preparation for a knee strike), the knees are turned in.

In a bow stance, the insubstantial back knee must not be straight or collapsed. There is a feeling of fullness in the W*ei Zhong* acupuncture point, which is situated behind the center of the knee.

COMMON MISTAKES:

Extending the knees too far forward—this happens when the knees go beyond the toes during horse stance or bow stance. In the attempt to maintain a lower posture, the lower-body strength is not sufficient to support the weight of the upper body. Ignorance of this aspect of body requirement can be a cause of this mistake.

Collapsing the knees—the knees are dropped forward. The substantial knee should point in the same direction as the foot. The insubstantial knee should not drop forward. The inside of the knee and the inside of the ankle need to be perpendicular to the ground.

Feet

Feet are the foundation of the body. In Chen Taijiquan the feet are used to push against the ground in order to create a rebounding energy. The Taiji classics say: "The *jing* is rooted in the feet, released through the legs, controlled by the waist and manifested through the hands." During practice, the toes grip the ground, the heels are against the ground, and the *Yongquan* points (below the ball of the foot and just on the toe half of the foot) are kept empty or insubstantial *(xu)*. These requirements make the foot full at the front and back but hollowed in the middle, which aids stability in movements and elasticity in power emission. Nevertheless, it is incorrect to deliberately contract and tense the foot to create a space. The foot is relaxed and natural, and not overly straight or artificially pressed down. The toes gripping the ground enable qi to go down to the root. The force emitted depends on the feet having a strong root.

It is the feet that distinguish fullness and emptiness. Weight is invariably unevenly distributed, mostly 60/40, but it can also be 70/30, 80/20 or even 90/10, with the exception of xu bu (empty stance), when the weight distribution is 100/0. The correct placement of a foot distributes even weight to the heel, toe, side and arch.

The weight-bearing foot should not move or rock about. When taking a step, use the inside heel to glide out and do not lift the toes. As the ankle joints move the feet, they are kept relaxed in order to co-ordinate with the feet.

COMMON MISTAKES:

Lifting the heel—this is known as "plucking the root" and often happens during fajing. When force is emitted to the left, the right heel may be lifted, resulting in reduced force as well as compromised balance.

Lifting the sides of the feet—causes stability to be lost.

Rocking the feet—the feet are not firmly planted on the ground. The foundation is absent and progress will not be made

Based on the correct principles and rules, practice the foundation until one is proficient. However, practice should be flexible, and adjusted to the different strengths and weaknesses of the practitioner, such as physical abilities and age. The overall guiding principle to follow is to be natural.

Essence of Chen Style Taijiquan

The Skill of *Fangsong*

The purpose of Taiji practice is to train internal energy in accordance with the correct principles. The basic Taiji principles are guidelines for *fangsong* (letting oneself relax and loosen up). This is the first difficult "gate" to pass through. Only then do you progress to learning the martial arts skill. Getting rid of tension in the whole body is the key. The first step, therefore, is to learn to loosen the body and to reduce tension. This requires repetitive practice, as the average person's disposition is at a more excited level than is required in Taijiquan.

A relaxed body is one where there is no tension in the muscles or friction in the joints. However, distinction must be made between being relaxed and being floppy. A floppy body is in negative tension. Relaxing does not mean making less effort. Being tense and being floppy are both incorrect in Taiji postures, since in both cases the flow of qi is blocked. Chen stylists liken this to a trampoline. The right tension in the springs of the trampoline enables a person to bounce on it. The more he pushes down, the higher he goes. If the trampoline is loose and soft, there is no rebounding power to gather height. If the spring is small and weak, one cannot fly. If the springs are too taut (hard), one is again stuck. Chen style stresses relaxed circular movements, requiring that circularity be sought through relaxation of the whole body, with outward-radial *jing* (*peng-jing*) as the basis.

There are four aspects of *fangsong*: Mind, Extension/Expansion, Sinking, and Pliancy.

Mind—The unity of body and mind is the key to achieving relaxation. One must quiet and relax the mind. When the mind is calm, *yi* (intent/consciousness) surfaces. One can then concentrate and focus the *yi*. Conversely, if the mind is not relaxed and calm, the *yi* is scattered, and this will have a reaction in the body. This follows the Taiji principles of yang arising from yin. The body is viewed as yang and the mind as yin. This mind-body relationship is described in the Chen family poem:

Breathe slowly, the heart (mind) will become quiet;
From quietness of the heart you become relaxed.

A calm mind increases awareness, and a relaxed body promotes sensitivity. The combination of the two will eventually unite the body and the mind.

Extension/Expansion—After relaxing the mind, emphasis is placed upon the joints and tendons. Seventeenth-generation master Chen Fa-ke stressed the need to loosen up every single joint in the body. The nine primary joints to loosen are the wrists, elbows, shoulders, ankles, knees, hips, back, waist and neck. The benefits of loosening the joints include the stretching and extension of muscles and tonus associated with a particular joint; an "open gateway" to allow qi to flow through the body to the extremities; and improvement in the strength and flexibility of tendons within the joint. Therefore all the joints in the body, as well as muscles and tendons, should be loosened and stretched; this extension extends even to the fingertips.

However, care must be taken not to extend in a single direction, or the extension will evolve into rigidity. There should be an idea of expansion as well as extension. This involves spreading or opening out in every direction simultaneously. For this to happen, when practicing, every part of the body should have opposing energies, especially the inside. For example, if one part of the body goes up, another part must go down. Forty percent of the energy distribution goes above the waist, and sixty percent goes down below the waist. As the Taiji principle dictates, all movements must have opposing energies—up must have down, left should have right, etc. Concentrate on opening and extension to begin with. As one advances, one can train opposing energies, opening on the outside and closing on the inside and vice versa.

Another aspect of relaxation is **sinking**. This element requires the body's center of gravity, together with the internal qi, to sink. With the exception of the head *(dingjing)*, the other main joints of the body should sink. Sinking down gives stability to the lower body. A strong lower body increases upper-body freedom. Sinking down also prevents qi from rising to the upper body, so that a posture does not "float." When properly executed, sinking creates the quality of weightedness *(zong)*, which translates as heaviness. It is not hard or rigid, but is characterized by softness on the outside and strength on the inside. When pushing hands this comes across as a heavy bearing-down force.

Pliancy, or the ability to move with ease and agility, is another aspect of relaxation. Relaxation increases the range of motion in the joints. Chen Taiji's silk-reeling method opens up and enlivens individual joints as it spirals in sequential movements. They become smooth and free to move in all directions. The tendons and muscles enjoy the same benefit, thus increasing elasticity and springiness.

The Concept of Open and Close

The concept of open *(kai)* and close *(her)* is part of the fundamental skills of Chen Taijiquan. Contained within each movement is opening and closing. Throughout every movement, the practitioner must distinguish where and how to change from open to closed and vice versa. Chen Xin emphasized the importance of understanding the principles of opening and closing in his writing. For instance, in *Chen Style Taijiquan with Illustrations and Theory* he said, "Open and closed, empty and solid, these are the principles of boxing."

Opening movements can be defined as those whereby, using the principle of silk-reeling, internal energy is guided by the mind from the dantian to the extremities of the limbs. Closing movements are those in which internal energy is drawn back to the dantian. Closing is given the characteristics of yin, opening being yang. Just as the philosophical concepts of yin and yang are interchangeable, so too, opening and closing movements can alternate freely. Generally, in motion there is opening; in stillness, there is closing. Expanding is seen as opening, contracting as closing. Releasing energy is opening; gathering energy is closing. Wang Zhongyue's Taijiquan manuscript states:

> Taiji emerges from Wuji. It is the origin of movement and stillness, and the mother of Yin and Yang. In movement the principle is to open, and in stillness the principle is to close.

The concepts of open and close represent two ideas that cannot be separated. In the Taiji classics it is said that within closing there is opening, and within opening there is closing. Throughout every posture and movement open and closed are present. Where the top of a posture is open, the bottom must be closed. When opening the right side, the left is closed. Like yin and yang, neither can be present without the other. For instance, in the posture White Crane Spreads Its Wings (*Bai He Liang Che*), the top is characterized by opening, the bottom by closing, externally open and internally closed.

The Single Whip (*Dan Bian*) posture at first sight appears to be totally open, with the arms widely extended and the legs far apart. Closer examination, however, reveals that while the posture is open when considered from left to right, it is closed from top to bottom. Combining opening of the limbs with a strong closing energy towards the center, the practitioner is poised to respond in any of the four directions. This is reflected in a song about the Single Whip posture passed down through generations of Taijiquan students and masters in Chenjiagou:

FIGURE 3.5
Chen Xiaowang in 'Single Whip'

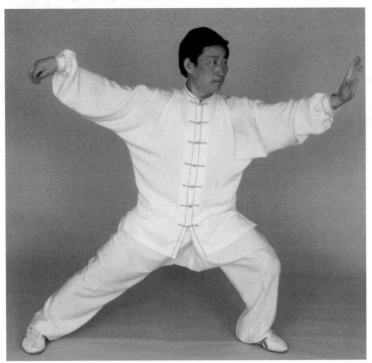

Single Whip strikes a majestic pose.
Unobstructed are the mai luo passageways.
The spirit perked, the form alert.
Arms like a snake span East to West.
Attack the head; the tail swings to defend.
Attack the tail; the head springs to counter.
Attack the center; head and tail jump to act.
Top and bottom and the four sides are thus guarded.
With the readiness of a stretched bow.
Where is the source of this ingenious posture?
Follow the backbone joints to its core.

Taijiquan, by adopting the principles of roundness and circularity, allows the practitioner to exhibit the characteristics of opening and closing simultaneously in any movement. Care must be taken when practicing opening and closing movements to concentrate upon internal work rather than action manifested externally. Considered from the perspective of practical application, roundness as a response to an opponent's action enables the practitioner to switch between open and closed at will, without communicating his reaction.

The Combination of Hard and Soft, Fast and Slow

A feature of Chen style Taijiquan is the combination of hard and soft movements, which are performed at a varying tempo, sometimes fast and sometimes slow. The combination of hard (*gang*) and soft (*rou*) is the essence of Chen Taiji, and the variant speed is necessary for practical reasons.

It is not easy to accomplish the right degree of *rou* and *gang*. *Gang* does not simply mean the use of strength or force, inasmuch as rou does not mean the absence of force. *Gang* is an elastic springy force (*dan huang jing*) that is generated through the waist in the process of silk-reeling movement. The root of "hard" movement is looseness and relaxation (*fangsong*). Taijiquan classics say: "From looseness one becomes soft; from accumulated softness hardness transpires; when hardness is expressed it returns to softness." Therefore, *gang* is the result of trained softness, and not of undisciplined stiff force or brute strength. It is manifested as heavy and sunken strength, as well as concealed internal hardness.

Rou is a pliable softness. The softness is not empty and lifeless but is full, firm and stable. *Rou* can only be achieved through consistent training following the right principles (see above section on The Skill of *Fangsong*). With this pliable softness, one will be able to follow, adhere and neutralize incoming force. It also allows one to move the whole body easily, without any obstruction or awkwardness. This creates the sensitivity required to discern threats and danger so that one can react instantly. According to Chen Zhaopei, "Pure *rou* without *gang* is soft boxing; pure *gang* without *rou* is stiff boxing. Only when there is a combination of *gang* and *rou* can one call it Taiji boxing."

When learning Taijiquan one should understand the implication behind the alternating fast and slow movements. Taijiquan is a self-defense art as well as a health-promoting exercise. Within the movements there are specific training methods and martial techniques. Therefore, each movement is designed for its practical use and contains a combination of fast and slow, hard and soft, open and closed, substantial and insubstantial, neutralizing and attacking.

Slow practice has the advantage of allowing one to concentrate on details; to check on accuracy of posture; to test stability and balance; to increase lower body strength; to co-ordinate internal and external movements; and to realize the circulation of qi throughout the body. All these are not possible if one performs the movements rapidly at the beginning. When proficient, movements should be a combination of slow and fast. Taijiquan classics state that "fast attacks require fast reactions; slow attacks require slow responses." Also "If the opponent does not move, I do not move. When he moves, I have already moved." The two statements show that Taiji skill requires fast reactions as well as slow, steady maneuvering. Slow practice is a training method and not the aim of Taijiquan. Training requires one's energy not to be dispersed when executing fast actions, and not to be broken when doing slow movements. Fast should not be stiff, and slow should not be feeble and floating (without root).

An Integrated Body: Internal and External Harmony

"Internal harmony" denotes the harmonizing of the *xin, yi, qi* and *li* (mind, intent, breath, and strength). This is sometimes referred to as the **three internal connections** or *li san he*, whereby *xin* and *yi* are connected, *yi* and *qi* are connected, and *qi* and *li* are connected. *Xin* is the chief and *yi* is the assistant. When *xin* decides, *yi* is activated. If the mind is disturbed, the intent will be scattered. This in turn leads to qi being diffused; it cannot be concentrated into *li*. Conversely, when qi settles, the intent will be focused, which in turn leads to the mind being calm. Therefore there is a close interconnection between *xin, yi, qi* and *li* that cannot be separated. These connections are difficult to achieve at the beginning. One starts with the help of visualization. For example, when executing a push in form practice, imagine that you are actually pushing an object (or an opponent) using mind intention. This will lead to qi moving, and *li* can be activated when needed.

Taijiquan, therefore, is a body and mind exercise. It requires that the whole body harmonize with the mind, intent and qi flow. When one part of the body is activated, the whole body follows. All movements are under the control of the mind. As the practitioner's body acquires the characteristic of being *song* (loose, relaxed and pliable), the mind becomes calm, focused and clear, with a spirit of alert attentiveness. When a person's movement is directed by yi or mind intent, then the qi follows and the body moves as a unified whole. Qi naturally goes to the appropriate places if the alignment and relaxation of the body are correct and not to blocking its natural flow. With correct practice over a period of time, an understanding develops of the internal firmness that lies behind the apparently slow and soft movements of Taijiquan. Externally it appears soft, but inside it is filled with strength.

The aim of Taiji practice is to involve the entire body so that in every movement the body works as an integrated system, not in isolated sections. In order to achieve this, one must be able to unite the internal connections with external connections and to synchronize upper and lower body movements. The whole body can be divided into three sections: upper, middle and lower body. These three sections must be connected and move as a single unit. The waist acts as the hub, co-ordinating the top and bottom. The waist is centralized to put in motion the arms and legs, followed by the hands and feet. If movements are done without connection among the three sections, then the center is lost and balance is upset easily. This requires careful study, persistent practice and laborious repetition. Impatience will not bring the desired outcome.

For the body to move as a single unit, there must be close coordination between its upper and lower parts. Taijiquan classics say that "from the feet to the legs to the waist and arms, all must be unified into an integrated whole," and "in movement everything moves, in stillness everything is still." If any one part of the body is not co-ordinated, then the whole body will be disordered and scattered. Using the waist as the axle linking the two halves, the upper limbs should be connected and the lower limbs co-ordinated. The requirements are that "when one opens, all are open; and when one closes all are closed." At the same time, there is open within closed and closed within open.

In the upper half of the body, coordination involves two aspects. The first is the coordination of both arms; the second is the synchronization of the arms and legs. Co-ordinating the arms involves the shoulders, the elbows and the hands. There should always be a link between the left and right sides. Between the arms, there are simultaneously opposing and combining forces, pulling them together as well as separating them. For example in the movement *Dan Bian* (Single Whip): when the left limb opens out in sequence, there should be a feeling of pulling apart from the right limb joint by joint. An example of the synchronization of arms and legs can be found in the *Qi Shi* (Preparing Form): when both arms are lifting up, the lower limbs regulate the movement. The shoulders, elbows and hands of the upper body are connected to the hips, knees and feet of the lower body. (This is known as the **three external connections** or *wai san he*.) There is a feeling of wanting to separate and yet being unable to separate; a feeling of wanting to unite and yet being unable to unite.

Similarly, the lower body, the two legs should be co-ordinated with each other, as well as synchronized with the upper limbs. When the top is insubstantial, the bottom is substantial and vice versa. Within emptiness there is fullness and within fullness there is emptiness. Coordination of both legs means that when the left leg spirals in *(shun-chan)*, the right should spiral out *(ni-chan)*, and when the right leg spirals in, the left leg spirals out; when one leg bends, the opposite leg stretches; when the left *kua* sits, the right *kua* relaxes, etc.

At the same time, when the top moves the lower body follows, and when the bottom moves the upper body follows. For example, if the leg moves, the hand follows, or if the hands lead, the legs follow. This principle can be clearly seen in the movement *Jin Gang Dao Dui* (Buddha's Warrior Attendant Pounds Mortar), where the lifting of the right knee is led by the right fist rising, and also in the movement *Bai He Liang Che* (White Crane Spreads Its Wings), during which the right arm opens upwards, drawing the left foot inwards.

The waist acts as the hub linking the two halves. Movement of the waist also contains two aspects: when the limbs move, the waist responds; when the waist moves, the limbs are activated. Therefore, when the arms move, the legs and the body (chest, waist and hips) move together, with qi moving to the top and bottom for a complete co-ordinated movement. For instance, in executing a *peng*: in the upper body the two arms *peng* upwards; the lower body sinks down on relaxed *kua*; the chest and waist unfold and open naturally; the upper body is insubstantial while the lower body is solid and substantial; above the waist qi circulates up; below the waist qi circulates down.

Another aspect of whole-body integration lies in Chen Taijiquan's sequential sectional method of movement. The Taijiquan classics say that "the whole body is linked section by section—do not let any part be broken." To illustrate this method: when *jing* is generated from the feet, it travels through the ankle, up the lower leg into the knee joint, then continues into the thigh to the *kua*. From the *kua* the waist is activated, sending movement through the back into the shoulder, then the elbow and finally the hand. Although sequential sectional movements are required, the degree of these movements is varied, as each action's demand on the various joints is different. Of the main joints of the body, those that are used most frequently and are the easiest to move are the wrist joints, and the least used is the torso. However, in Taiji practice, it is recommended that one reduce the wrist movement and increase the torso movement. As the teachers often say, "Practice Taiji with the body, not with the hands."

For sectional movement to be realized, the body is conveniently divided into sections and then subdivided. The body consists of three main sections: the outer/top section; the middle section; and the root/lower section. The upper limbs are the top section, the torso is the middle section, and the lower limbs are the root section. Each of these is further subdivided. In the upper limbs, the hands are the outer section, the elbow the middle section, and the shoulders the root section. In the body, the head is the upper section, the waist the middle section, and the abdomen the root section. In the lower limbs, the foot is the outer section, the knee the middle section, and the *kua* the root section. These make up the nine major sections of the body. The upper sections are involved with *shoufa* (hand techniques) and the lower sections with *bufa* (footwork and leg techniques).

There are also "eighteen balls," denoting the main joints of the body. These are: two shoulders, two elbows, two wrists, two kuas, two knees, two ankles, two hips/buttocks, neck, chest, waist, and abdomen. Whole-body movement is facilitated by the twining and spiralling action of the eighteen balls, moving through each section in strict sequence.

These fundamentals need to be understood so that the method can be practiced with ease and skill. There should be no irregularities in movement

(e.g. rising up and down, shaking the head) unless they are integral aspects of the form. All movements are expressed in the same sequence of equilibrium.

The Five Bows

A bow is defined in the *Oxford English Dictionary* as a "weapon for shooting arrows, a strip of flexible wood or other material held in a bent position when in use, by a string stretched between its two ends." The bow's characteristic of developing stretching power via two opposing forces is often used to explain the internal power mechanics of Taijiquan. The bow comprises both yin and yang aspects. Insufficient strength when drawing back the string, and there will be no energy with which to propel the arrow. Too much strength, and the bow will break. In the Taijiquan postures, a relationship exists between the curved shape of the full side and the force point of the empty side. To create stretching power within the body, the practitioner must embrace the outside (yang) while supporting the inside (yin).

Noted Taijiquan historian Gu Liuxin compares the body requirements of Chen Taijiquan to "one body holding five bows." Taijiquan requires all parts of the body to be curved. Although many bow forms are present, Gu Liuxin suggests that there are five major ones: the body represents one bow; the two arms represent two bows; and the final two bows are represented by the two legs. Each of the bows has the capacity to store and emit force. When combined, this forms the basis for focused whole-body *jing*, as the collective force of the entire body is emitted through one point.

The "body bow" is formed by linking the body's head and trunk. Two opposing pulling forces are present—at the top of the neck (*Anmen* at the first neck bone) and the base of the spine (*Changqiang* point). By suspending the top of the head and tucking in the buttocks while relaxing the waist, these two points are pulled apart, storing energy in the spine. The *Anmen* point becomes insubstantial; the center of the back at the *Dazui* point is raised slightly, while the tailbone is tucked in and substantial. Concentrating upon tucking in the chin, holding the neck erect but relaxed, tucking the hips in and storing the chest leads the back to curve inwards, and the chest to strengthen the outside.

Regardless of what movement is being performed, Taijiquan requires the practitioner to straighten the back, sink the elbows and seat the wrists. When considered together, both arms stretch out to form the shape of a bow. In extending outwards from the center, the two wrists provide opposing forces and are linked together like a bowstring. Taken individually, each arm can be seen as a bow in its own right. The elbow corresponds to the middle of the bow, where one would hold before pulling back the drawstring with the other hand. Intention is focused on the elbow joint to make sure that it remains relaxed, sunken and aimed. The wrist and clavicle correspond to the two ends of the bow. If the two directional pulling forces are to be created then both ends must be firm and steady. Flexibility of the arm is a result of seating the wrist and ensuring that the clavicle is steady so that it does not lean or shake. The stability of the clavicle determines the stability and movement direction of the arm.

The two legs assume a bow shape by sinking the body down, rounding the crotch, opening the upper legs and pulling the knees inwards slightly. Viewed together, the two legs are shaped like a bow, with the ankles linked together like a bowstring. Considering each leg separately, the knee can be seen as the center of the bow, the ends being the *kua* and the heel. To ready the leg bow, the knee is pushed forward slightly without being allowed to collapse. At the same time, the kua relaxes, sinks down and sits slightly back, and the heel is pressed down firmly into the ground. After pressing down the heel, energy is transmitted out from the ground in a spiral movement. At all times an opposing force is present. This is in line with Taijiquan's requirement of moving down before moving up, left before right, etc.

If the internal and external are to be co-ordinated, all five bows must be present. This is true whether one is practicing the hand form, push hands or weapons. Of the five bows, the body bow is primary, the arm and leg bows secondary. Using the waist as the hub, the upper body is connected by the two arms, the lower body by the two legs. When all the requirements are met and the upper and lower body are connected, the middle naturally follows. At all times the practitioner should maintain these five bows. In this way his body will be flexible and responsive in every direction. As the Taiji classics say: "All eight directions are strong." In a verse written by Chen Zhongsheng, father of Chen Xin, he captures the essence of Taijiquan, like an archer about to release an arrow:

Light like scattered flowers,
Solid like tempered metal.
Competing with the tiger for ferocity,
Challenging the eagle for speed.
In movement it is like a flowing river,
In stillness it is like a solid mountain,
The spirit concentrated at the brink before emitting.

Zhong Ding (Central Equilibrium)

*While standing, the body is centered and comfortable,
supported in all eight directions.*

*The tailbone centered, the spirit rises to the crown.
From top to bottom one straight line.*

The correct execution of the Chen form involves the development of central equilibrium, or *zhong ding*. In the preceding verses, Chen Xin stresses the importance of maintaining a centrally balanced position when practicing Taijiquan. Zhong ding is usually considered to be the most essential of the thirteen basic skills of Taijiquan. The separation from stillness to the yin-yang polarity is essential to the other twelve skills. This follows the often-quoted Taiji theory, which states that *wuji* gives birth to Taiji. Or that stillness and non-action is the source of the yin-yang polarity, which is characterized by movement and action. Failing to establish central equilibrium prevents the practitioner from differentiating between the opposites of open and closed, empty and solid, or substantial and insubstantial.

Breathing

By combining external martial techniques with the traditional methods of *daoyin* (guiding qi) and *tu-na* (deep breathing exercises originating from the dantian), Chen Wangting created a system characterized by the integration of consciousness, movement and breathing. An old Taijiquan verse suggests: "On the outside you exercise the tendons, skin and bones; on the inside you train the breathing." The various training methods such as the hand and weapons forms, silk-reeling exercises, push hands, etc., with their use of whole-body twining and spiralling movements, certainly train the body. Internally, the use of deep, regulated, natural breathing massages the internal organs, ensuring that there is a smooth flow of blood and qi throughout the body.

Taijiquan uses two types of breathing pattern, commonly referred to as "normal" and "reverse" breathing. When normal breathing is being employed, the stomach expands as the practitioner inhales and contracts as he exhales. With reverse breathing, the opposite is true. First and foremost, breathing should be natural. The breathing method of Taijiquan follows certain principles, such as: inhaling when "closing" or bringing in, and exhaling when "opening" or extending; inhaling when storing or gathering energy, exhaling when emitting energy; inhaling when rising up, exhaling when dropping down. However, even within these requirements breathing may vary depending upon the circumstance.

For instance, when releasing power the practitioner reverts to reverse breathing, whereby the abdomen contracts during inhalation and is distended during exhalation. Chen style Taijiquan utilizes reverse breathing as a means of increasing martial power. Each striking movement is characterized by an exhalation, an expansion of the abdomen, and a sensation of qi sinking down to the dantian. Exhaling rapidly to increase power is a feature shared with many other Chinese martial arts. Expanding the abdomen and sinking qi downwards facilitate balance and stability.

Even when doing *fajing*, the breathing must be spontaneous and natural. If the breath has to be forced then it is unnatural and detrimental to health. In fact, reversed breathing is used unconsciously whenever a person makes a sudden, violent effort, even if they are completely unaware of it. Just as a person could not inhale while pushing a car, one cannot inhale when performing *fajing*.

Above all, the body must not be deprived of its natural need for air just to accommodate a breathing formula. Forcing one's breathing can only result in a breathing pattern that is interrupted and not smooth, blocking the flow of internal energy and hindering vitality and spirit. A common mistake is to put too much emphasis on trying to control the breath during movement. Left to itself, the body will adjust the breathing to accommodate the body's requirements. For example, if a person engages in strenuous activity such as running or swimming, as they put in greater effort, the breath naturally responds to the body's needs. As more demands are placed on the body many details may be forgotten, but never breathing.

The importance of naturalness and spontaneity (*zi ran*) in breathing cannot be overemphasized. The Chinese term *zi ran* literally means "own nature"—that which occurs by following the rules of its own character. With time and practice, the student's movement should reach a higher standard and begin to approach the correct principles of how to open and close, etc. With increasing refinement of movement, the body will naturally regulate itself to follow the correct method of breathing.

Chen Xiaowang's Five Levels of Skill

Learning Taijiquan can be compared to going to school to educate oneself. Progressing from primary to university level, one gradually gathers more and more knowledge. Without the foundation gleaned from primary and secondary education, one will not be able to follow the curriculum of the university level. To learn Taijiquan one also needs a gradual and systematic progression, from the elementary to the advanced level. If one goes against this tenet he will not succeed. There are no shortcuts.

The whole process of learning Taijiquan, from the beginning to full accomplishment, can be separated into five stages or levels of skill (*gong fu*). There are objective standards for each, indicating the level of skill, with the fifth level being the highest. The standard and requirements for each level are described in the following sections. It is hoped that with these descriptions, Taijiquan enthusiasts will be able to assess their own current level of attainment. They will also know what they need to learn in order to advance systematically.

The First Level of Skill

Taijiquan requires the body to be upright, head lifted as if pulled from the crown, shoulders relaxed and elbows sunk, chest stored and waist folded, crotch opened and knees bent, leading the inner energy to sink down to the dantian. A beginner may not be able to master all these important points immediately. However, he must aim to be accurate in posture in terms of direction, angle, position and the movement paths of the arms and legs. At this level, one need not place too much emphasis on the requirements for different parts of the body: appropriate simplifications are acceptable. For example, for the head and the upper body, it is sufficient for the head and body to be kept naturally upright and not leaning forward or backward, left or right. Just like learning to write Chinese characters, at the beginning one need only make sure that the strokes are correct.

When initially practicing Taijiquan, the body as well as movements will appear stiff—*"externally solid but internally empty."* There will be hard hitting, ramming, abrupt rising and falling. The *jing* (force) will be broken or resistant. These are all common phenomena. If one is persistent and practises every day, proficiency in the form will be achievable within half a year. With refinements in one's postures, qi can gradually be driven by external movements to move within the body and limbs. The first level of skill thus begins with refining the postures to gradually be able to detect and understand *jing*.

Martial application within the first level is very limited. This is because actions are not well co-ordinated and synchronized. The postures are not yet correct. The *jing* produced may be stiff, broken, and either too strong or too lax. The form may appear hollow and angular. One may feel the internal energy but not be able to channel it as a whole to every part of the body. Consequently one is not able to harness the force or *jing* from the feet, through the legs, and discharge it through the control of the waist. Instead a beginner can only produce broken *jing* that surges from one section of the body to another. The first-level skill, therefore, is insufficient for martial applications. If one were to test one's skill on someone who does not know martial arts, to a certain extent one may appear nimble. Although the applications may not have been mastered, by knowing how to lead away, one may occasionally be able to throw off an opponent. However, body balance may not be maintained.

This situation is termed **"One Yin and Nine Yang—Top Heavy Staff"** or *Yi Yin Jiu Yang Gen Tou Guen.*

What are yin and yang? In the context of practicing Taijiquan, emptiness is yin, solidity is yang; close is yin, open is yang; softness is yin, hardness is yang. Yin and yang are the unity of opposites, one incomplete without the other, yet mutually interchangeable. If a maximum of ten were assigned to measure them, then an equal balance of five yin and five yang would indicate ultimate success. The first level, One Yin and Nine Yang, demonstrates skill that is more hard than soft, and there is an imbalance. The learner is not yet able to complement hard with soft and to command the application with ease. Therefore, at this stage the pursuit of the applications aspect of postures is not necessary.

The Second Level of Skill

The second level of skill involves further reducing shortcomings such as stiff internal and external *jing* while practicing the form; and uncoordinated movements due to over- or under-exertion of force. This is to ensure that the qi/internal energy moves in the body in accordance with the requirements of each movement. Eventually, this will lead to a smooth flow of internal qi in the body that coordinates with external movements.

After acquiring the first level of skill, one should be familiar with the movements, practice according to the preliminary requirements, and feel the movement of internal qi. However, one is not yet able to control the flow of qi in the body. There are two reasons for this: firstly, the specific requirements for each part of the body and their coordination have not been accurately mastered. For example, storing/relaxing the chest too much leads to the back hunching; loosening the waist too much leads to the chest and buttocks protruding. One must strictly ensure that the body requirements are met and strive to resolve any contradictions. This will ensure that each part of the body moves in unison. The whole body will then harmonize and unite, both internally and externally. (Internal harmony—heart and mind; internal energy and strength; tendons and bones. External harmony—hands and feet; elbows and knees; shoulders and hips.) Simultaneously, there should be an equal and opposing energy. Closing and opening movements come together and complement each other.

Secondly, it may be difficult to control different parts of the body all at once. Sometimes one part of the body moves faster than the rest, resulting in resistive force. Another part of the body may move too slowly, thereby losing energy. Both contradict the principles of Taijiquan. No movement in Chen style Taijiquan should deviate from the silk-reeling energy or *chan-ssu-jing*. According to the theory of Taijiquan, "the *chan-ssu-jing* originates from the kidneys and is found in every part of the body at all times." In the process of learning Taijiquan, the silk-reeling method (i.e., the twining and spiralling method of movement) and the silk-reeling energy (i.e., the inner force produced from the reeling-silk method of movement) need to be properly mastered through keeping the shoulders and elbows relaxed, as well as the chest and waist, crotch and knees, using the waist as an axis to move every part of the body. When rotating the hands inwards, the hands lead the elbows, which lead the shoulders, which in turn lead the waist (the part of the waist corresponding to the side that is being moved—in actual fact the waist is still the axis). When the hand rotates out, the waist moves the shoulders, which move the elbows, and the elbows in turn move the hands. From an external point of view, looking at the upper half of the body, the wrists and arms appear to be gyrating. In the lower part of the body, the ankles and the legs appear to be rotating. In the trunk, the waist and back appear to be turning. Combining the three parts, one should visualize rotating in space, a curve that originates from the legs, with the center at the waist and ends at the fingers. In practicing the form, if a particular movement feels awkward, then use *chan-ssu-jing's* sequence of flow as the guideline for adjusting the body in order to achieve harmony of movement. In this way, errors can be corrected. Therefore, while paying attention to the requirements for each part of the body in order to achieve whole-body coordination, the mastering of the principles of silk-reeling method and silk-reeling energy is a method by which to resolve contradictions and for to correct oneself during practice in the second level of skill.

In the first level of skill, one begins with learning the form, and when the form becomes familiar, a learner will start to feel the

FIGURE 3.6
Chen Xiaowang adjusting Davidine Sim's posture

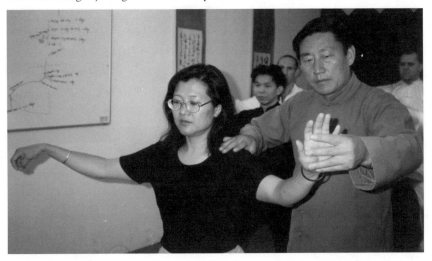

movement of internal qi within the body. The interest level is high, and there is seldom boredom. However, upon entering the second level, there may be a feeling of staleness, and very often certain important points may not yet be fully understood. Because of inaccuracies, movements during practice may be awkward, or perhaps the movements can be performed smoothly, and force expressed with much vigor, but during push hands no skill can be applied. As a result, one may soon feel discouraged and suffer loss of confidence, or simply abandon the practice altogether. Only through persistent practice and strict adherence to correct principles can one achieve a stage where one is able to produce just the right amount of *jing*, change at will, and rotate with ease. One has to train hard in form practice so that the body becomes one single unit, which enables one movement activating all movements.

There is a common saying: "If the principle is not clearly understood, consult a teacher. If the way is not clearly visible, seek the help of friends." When the principles as well as the methods are clearly understood, with constant practice success will eventually prevail. The Taijiquan classics state, "Everybody can possess the ultimate, if only one works diligently." Also: "if one is persistent, eventually he will achieve a sudden breakthrough." Generally it takes about four years to attain the second level of skill. When one reaches the stage at which qi saturates the whole body, then sudden realization transpires. One is then filled with confidence and enthusiasm and the strong urge to go on practicing.

During the early part of the second level, the martial ability and application are similar to that of the first level. It is not sufficient for practical usage. At the end of the second level approaching the third level, the martial ability is only applicable to a certain extent. The next paragraph describes the martial ability that should be attainable mid-way through the second level (in the third, fourth and fifth levels, description also refers to the mid-way stage).

Push hands and form practice are inseparable. Whatever shortcomings one has in the form will certainly show up as weaknesses during push hands, giving an opponent the opportunity to take advantage. Therefore, Taijiquan requires the whole body to move together, devoid of any unnecessary movements. Push hands requires one "to pay attention to and differentiate between *peng-lu-ji-an;* a good coordination in the upper and lower body will prevent an opponent from entering; no matter how hard he attacks, four ounces can deflect a thousand pounds." The second level of skill aims to achieve saturation of qi throughout the body, correction of body movements, and the flow of qi in sequence to all joints and sections of the body. The process of adjusting body postures often causes unnecessary and uncoordinated movements. As a result, when doing push hands one is unable to apply martial technique at will. The opponent will exploit these weaknesses, like leading one to commit to wrong technique such as resisting with stiff force or a collapsed frame. An opponent's advances will not allow time for one to make the necessary adjustments to the body movements. Instead, all shortcomings will be used to his advantage, making one lose balance, or compelling one to step back in order to ward off the attack. On occasions when an opponent advances with less force and at a slower speed, one may have the time and opportunity to make adjustments and fend off an attack successfully. At the second level of skill, therefore, much effort is required to make an attack or to block an attack. Very often it is a case of attacking first to gain advantage. One is unable to "forget oneself and follow others" or to change tactics at will in response to a situation. Diversion techniques may work, but errors such as too much or too little force are common. The techniques of *peng-lu-ji-an* cannot be executed.

This level is **"Two Yin and Eight Yang—An Undisciplined New Hand"** or *Er Yin Ba Yang Shi San Shou* .

The Third Level of Skill

"If you wish to do well in your quan *[form], you must train to make the circle smaller."* The stages of practicing Chen style Taijiquan involve

reducing the circle from big to medium to small, and eventually to no circle. "Circle" does not refer to the route of movement of the limbs, but rather to the path of internal qi circulation. The third level of skill is the transition from big circle to medium circle.

Taijiquan classics state that the *"yi and qi are superior to the form."* When practicing Taiji one should place emphasis on using the *yi* (mind/consciousness). At the first level of skill, one's mind and concentration are mainly on learning and mastering the external forms. During the second level, one concentrates on eliminating the contradiction of internal and external movements, by adjustments of the body. At the third level, the internal energy is understood and flows smoothly. What is required is the use of *yi* and not *li* (stiff force). Movements should be light but not flaccid, weighted but not stiff. There is inner strength within soft external movements, with strong force implied in soft movements. The body is well co-ordinated and devoid of any irregular movements. Nevertheless, one should avoid paying attention to qi flow only and neglecting the external motions. Otherwise, one would appear vague and distracted. Qi not only fails to circulate smoothly, but may stagnate or become dispersed. As stated in the Taijiquan classics: "Attention should be on the spirit and not just qi; with too much emphasis on qi there will be stagnation."

In the first and second level, although one masters the external form, the internal and external movements are not yet synchronized. Due to stiffness or stagnation in a movement, inhalation may be restricted. Or, due to lack of coordination of internal and external movements, exhalation may be incomplete. Therefore, only natural breathing is recommended. Upon entering the third level of skill, however, some obvious actions will naturally and correctly synchronize with the breathing as internal and external movements become better coordinated. For more subtle, complex and faster actions, it is necessary to consciously co-ordinate the breathing until breath and action gradually and naturally harmonize.

The third level of skill basically involves mastering the internal and external requirements of Chen style Taijiquan, as well as movement principles. When one has the ability to correct one's own shortcomings, and to move with ease as well as to summon sufficient internal qi, then one is ready to move a step further towards the understanding and application of the combat skill implicit in each posture. To this end, one needs to practice push hands; check on the forms; understand the internal force *(jing)*; and learn how to express the force *(fajing)* as well as how to neutralize the force *(hua-jing)*. If one is able to withstand confrontational pushhands, then it is an indication that one has understood the underlying Taiji principles. Continuous training will lead to increased confidence. At this point one can step up one's training and bring in supplementary training such as shaking the long pole; practicing with weapons such as the sabre, spear, sword, and staff; and doing single-posture training such as *fajing*. Training in this manner for two years, one can generally advance into the fourth level of skill.

During the third level, there is qi circulation throughout, and movements are better co-ordinated. However, the internal qi is still not strong enough to establish harmony of muscle movements with functioning of the internal organs. One may be able to achieve internal and external unity while practicing alone without external disturbances. During confrontational push hands, if an advance is not forceful or too fast, one may be able to follow the opponent; change technique as situation dictates; turn opportunity to one's advantage; entice into emptiness; evade danger and attack weak points; and maneuver and neutralize at will and with ease. However, on encountering an opponent of better skill, one will feel that one's *peng* (warding) energy is insufficient and may experience a feeling of being compressed (which will probably destroy a posture that should be neither leaning nor declining, and supported in all directions). One will be unable to maneuver at will, and to emulate the Taijiquan classics that require one to *"strike with hands that are invisible to the opponent; once visible cannot go."* Both neutralizing and emitting skills feel awkward and require much effort.

This level of skill is **Three Yin and Seven Yang—Still on the Hard Side**, *San Yin Qi Yang Yu Jien Ying*.

The Fourth Level of Skill

The fourth level requires the circle to be further reduced from medium to small. This is the stage nearing accomplishment and thus demonstrates a high level of proficiency. One has mastered the effective method of training; the movement principles; the martial/combat meaning in each posture; the smooth circulation of internal qi; and harmony of actions with breathing. During training, however, it is necessary to imagine facing an opponent with each step and each action. One has to imagine being surrounded by enemies. For each posture of each form, each part of the body must be linked in continuous movements, so that the whole body moves as a single unit. The upper and lower parts of the body are connected, controlled at the waist and driven by continuous qi flow. When practicing the form, *"nobody is there but imagine somebody is there."* In actual confrontation, one should be courageous but cautious, acting as if *"nobody is there when somebody is there."* Training content at this level is similar to that of the third level (like form and weapons). With perseverance, the fifth level of skill can generally be reached in three years.

In terms of martial skill there are significant differences between the third and fourth level. The third level achieves ability to neutralize the opponent's force and to rid contradictions in one's own movements, in order to be able to play an active role and force the opponent into passivity. At the fourth level of skill one can neutralize as well as emit force. That is due to the fact that one has ample internal *jing*; ease of *yi* and *qi* exchange; and a consolidated system of body movements. During push hands, the opponent's attack does not pose a big threat. When in contact with an opponent, one can change maneuvers instantly and easily neutralize or deflect incoming force. Thus, special characteristics are developed such as following an opponent's movements while being flexible; neither losing nor resisting; internal attunement; staying ahead of the opponent's intentions; conciseness of movement; emitting force with precision; and hitting targets accurately.

This is described as **Four Yin and Six Yang—Akin to a Good Hand**, *Si Yin Liu Yang Lei Hao Shou*.

The Fifth Level of Skill

The fifth level of skill is the stage in which one moves from small circle to invisible circle, from visible movements to undetectable form. Taijiquan classics say: *"Qi flowing without interruption, the cosmic qi blending with natural internal qi, moving from a form to one without trace, one realizes how remarkable nature is."* During the fifth level of skill, movements are smooth and flexible, internal strength abounds, but it is still necessary to strive for the best. Each day's training will bring new achievement, until the body is totally free of constraints, with limitless possibilities for change. The internal alternation of substantial and insubstantial is not discernible outside. Only then is the fifth level attained.

From the point of view of martial skill, at this level the *gang* (hard) complements the *rou* (soft). Movements are relaxed, dynamic, springy and elastic. Taiji principles are evident in every part of the body and every movement. Reactions are precise and rapid. Sensitive to external stimuli, any part of the body can be used for attack, wherever it comes into contact with an opponent. There must be a constant interchange between expressing force and conserving energy, with a solid stance that is supported on all sides. Therefore, *"only the one who exhibits five yin and five yang, without discrepancies in the yin and yang, is acknowledged as a true master. A true master's every move is Taiji, with every move indiscernible."*

The fifth level, therefore, is **Five Yin and Five Yang—A True Master**, *Wu Yin Wu Yang Cheng Miao Shou*.

After completing the fifth level of skill, there is good control of the mind and emotions, and good coordination of muscular contraction and relaxation, as well as the functioning of the internal organs. Sudden attacks will not disrupt these harmonies, as one is fully adaptable. Even so, one should continue to pursue further knowledge so as to achieve the ultimate.

 Development in science is boundless, as is the study of Taijiquan. Its wonder can never be expended in a lifetime.

Unabridged translation from Chen Xiaowang's
Wu Chen Gongfu

The task of developing correct habits is a gradual process. This task is often painstaking and arduous. The first step is to understand and manage basic body movements and not be impatient for the more complex techniques.

Taijiquan requires the body to be used in a unique disciplined way. The first training requirement must be to discard old habits, to approach with an "empty cup"—if your cup is full of your own tea, there will be no room for the flavor of new tea. In other words, one must put aside what one has learned previously so that the mind is clear and open to receive new information without bias and preconception.

According to Chen Fa-ke, those who study Taijiquan should not only understand the theories *(li)* in their mind; they need to train the methods *(fa)* into their body. They should understand why but it is just as important to understand how—*"how much you accomplish depends entirely on how much effort you put in."*

Chen Xin writes: "All that idle talk does is to create a tide of black ink; actually putting it into practice is the real thing."

All practice should be "according to the rules" *(an zhe gui ju)*.

Common Acupuncture Points in Chen Style Taijiquan

I. *Baihui* (DU20)

Situated at the crown of the head. This point should be lightly lift-ed; the head feels as if it is suspended by a string attached to this point. All yang meridians meet here.

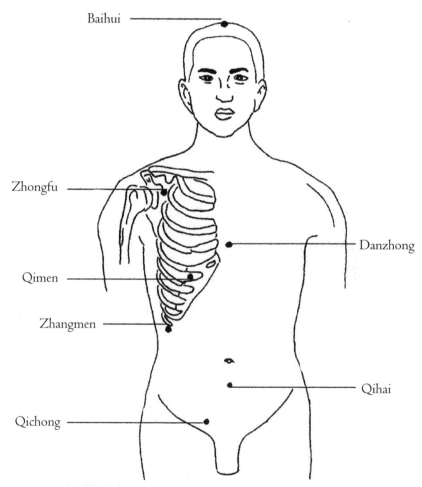

FIGURE 3.7
Common Acupuncture points in Chen Taijiquan—Front View

2. Jianjing (GB21)

Situated in the depression on the top of each shoulder, forming a vertical line with the nipple. Level the two shoulders in the process of relaxing them. Keep the *Jianjing* level with the *Dadui points* (see below). Do not use force to deep them level, whether in motion or in stillness. If the shoulders are raised qi floats and power is lost. With correct alignment, the qi rises to the *Baihui* and sinks down to the *Yongquan* in the feet.

3. Zhongfu (LU1)

Located on the lateral part of the thoracic wall, on the level of the first intercostal space. Relaxing this point helps relax the clavicles (collar bones), and therefore the shoulders.

4. Danzhong (RN17)

On the chest at the midpoint of the line connecting both nipples. Mind intent is focused on this point during execution of *an* (press down).

5. Qimen (LR14)

Located on the chest, directly below the nipple on the sixth inter-costal space. When qi goes through this point, the cyclic door will be opened to facilitate the cycle of qi flow.

6. Zhangmen (LR13)

On the lateral side of the abdomen, below the free end of the eleventh rib. Mind focus and relaxation on this point enables qi to travel down from the chest. Obstruction at this point causes tightness in the chest.

7. Qichong (ST30)

Slightly above the inguinal crease (*kua*). Relax the *kua* to let qi go through this point. When qi goes down the inner thigh into the legs, one feels the weight sinking down to the feet, making the lower body weighted and stable.

8. *Quchi* (LI11)

With the elbow flexed, the point is situated at the lateral end of the crease. Regardless of posture, the elbow joints are kept slightly arced, and pulling down towards the *Yongquan*. Mentally focus the internal energy from the *Quchi* along the arms to the wrists and then to the hands, where power can be issued.

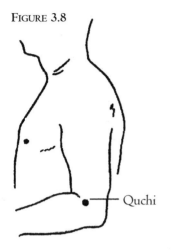

FIGURE 3.8

Quchi

9. *Laogong* (PC8)

Located at the center of the palm, at the place where the tip of the fourth finger lands when it is flexed. The *Laogong* point is kept insubstantial when practicing Taiji. This results in a feeling of qi being retained within the palm and internal power extended out. Whether the hands are open or closed (as in making a fist) the *Laogong* should remain insubstantial, so the internal power reaches the inside of the fingers.

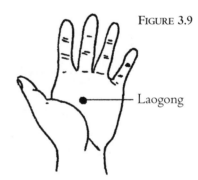

FIGURE 3.9

Laogong

10. *Qihai* (RN6)

One and a half inches (or three finger widths) below the umbilicus. The dantian is located within this point. Qi is stored here before being directed out to various parts of the body. The muscles in this area should not be tense. A feeling of fullness and warmth is felt when qi is abundant.

11. *Huiyin* (RN1)

Located between the genitalia and the anus. This point is gently lifted during Taiji practice, along with the *Baihui* at the top of the head. This keeps the lower back firm and strong.

12. *Changqiang* (DU1)

Below the top of the coccyx, at the midpoint of the line connecting the end of the coccyx and anus. The *Changqiang* is kept relaxed and points downwards. By keeping the direction of this point and the nose in a straight line, correct body alignment and whole-body movement can be achieved.

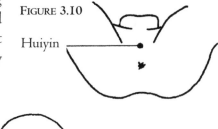

FIGURE 3.10

Huiyin

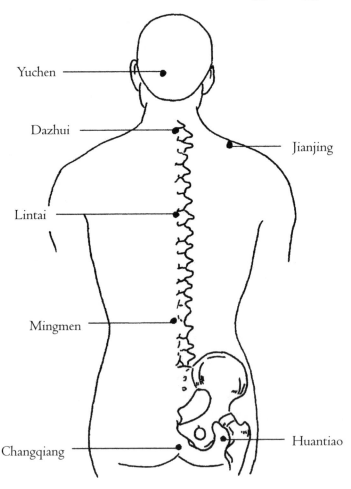

FIGURE 3.11
Common Acupuncture points in Chen Taijiquan—Rear View

13. *Mingmen* (DU4)
Located on the lower back below the second lumbar vertebra. When the whole chest is relaxed and qi is sunk down to the dantian, the *Mingmen* will naturally protrude slightly. This area is the mainstay of all Taiji movements and power emission, and is therefore a very significant point in Chen style Taijiquan.

14. *Dadui* (DU14)
On the middle upper back, in the depression below the seventh cervical vertebra, this point lines up with the *Jianjing* to maintain correct shoulder alignment.

15. *Jiaji/Lintai* (DU10)
On the back below the sixth thoracic vertebra. Slightly expand this point to keep the arms rounded in front of the body. Qi is directed from this point outwards in *ji* (squeeze) action, and when emptying to the right.

16. *Yuchen* (BL9)
On the back of the head where the base of the skull connects with the top of the neck. Relaxing this point helps the neck muscles relax, letting qi travel upwards to the *Baihui* and downwards to the dantian. Also helps clear the mind.

17. *Weizhong* (BL40)
Situated at the midpoint of the popliteal crease at the back of the knee. This point should be kept full in all postures, with the back of the knee holding energy. When this point is allowed to slacken, the knee joints become weak and the leg will lose its support.

18. *Huantiao* (GB30)
Huantiao is located on the hip joint in the depression near the greater trochanter. When the upper body is relaxed and *Weizhong* kept full, with the whole body in correct alignment, the *Huantiao* will feel full and will turn outward. Qi rushes down the *Qichong*

through the inner thigh and "jumps" up through the outer thigh at the *Huantiao* point. Qi connections between the legs and the trunk are maintained through this point.

Figure 3.12

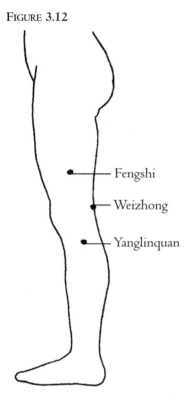

19. *Fengshi* (GB31)
Located on the side of the thigh at the spot touched by the middle finger when standing straight with the arms hanging freely. This point is touched and qi is stimulated during *Wuji* stance, or at the beginning of the Taiji routine (*Qishe*).

20. *Yanglinquan* (GB24)
Located on the side of the knee, in the depression at the head of the fibula, this point is connected with the middle section of the lower limb (just as Quchi is to the middle section of the upper limb).

21. *Yongquan* (KI1)
Located on the sole of the foot, in the depression at the center when the foot and toes are flexed, the *Yongquan* point should be kept insubstantial and not be pressed down into the ground when standing. When placing the foot, weight should be distributed throughout the foot equally, not leaning towards the toes, nor the heels, nor the sides.

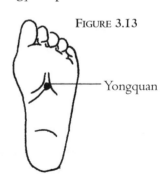

Figure 3.13

Yongquan

In Chen style Taijiquan the acupuncture points are important in relation to movements. Different postures require various coordinations of the muscles. The acupuncture points and channels particular to the different muscles are stimulated and activated because qi in the body communicates through them. At the same time, focusing the mind on the related points enables the muscle group as well as qi movement to respond in a particular manner.

The acupuncture points also act as "boundaries," helping to keep qi contained. Using them as starting and finishing points, one is able to keep internal qi circulation and external movements within the desired perimeter.

Qi Storage: Dantian and the Internal Organs

"Dantian" means, literally, the elixir *(dan)* field *(tian)*. It is located in the lower abdomen, midway between the navel and the pubic bone, and is the most important center in the body, frequently referred to in Taijiquan practice. It is the body's center of gravity as well as the energy center. The dantian stores qi and drives it throughout the body. By concentrating on this point, one learns to harvest, cultivate and nourish qi energy, and also to direct it to different parts of the body. The dantian is maintained as the body's centre throughout Taijiquan practice.

Qi is also stored in the internal organs, which are arranged into yin and yang organs. Yin organs, known as *Zang*, consist of the heart, liver, spleen, kidneys and lungs. The yang organs, known as *Fu*, are the stomach, large intestine, small intestine, bladder and gall bladder. According to Chinese theory, *Zang* are the organs that store essential substances for the body's use. *Fu* do not store substances but eliminate them; they are essentially hollow.

The emphasis on holding the body without tension in Taijiquan helps to eliminate or reduce stress in the areas where the internal organs are situated. The spiral twining movements of Chen style Taijiquan gently massage the internal organs, keeping them in optimum health to carry out their functions.

Ren Mai and Du Mai

These two main energy channels are located at the front and back of the body. The front channel is called *Ren Mai*, or Conception Channel. It contains the yin circulation and starts from the base of the mouth, extending down the center of the front body to the *Huiyin* point between the legs. The channel at the back is called *Du Mai*, or Governing Channel. This channel starts from the *Huiyin* point, runs along the spinal column from the coccyx up through the neck and over the top of the head, to end at the roof of the mouth. It contains the most important yang circulation. The two channels are not connected at the top, and the circuit needs to be completed by placing the tongue at the roof of the mouth. This circuit is known as the Small Heavenly Circulation *(Xiao Zhou Tian)*. These two channels aid the flow of yin and yang energies in the body, and help to regulate qi circulation of the internal organs. For qi to circulate throughout the body, the main channels must have a strong flow in order to be able to reach the lesser tributaries (the organ meridians). When qi circulates to the entire body, it is known as the Great Heavenly Circulation *(Da Zhou Tian)*.

Dai Mai and Chung Mai

Dai Mai or the Belt Channel, as the name implies, encircles the body at the waist. It is responsible for qi's horizontal balance. In the absence of this balance, the body's center is lost. When qi circulation is complete in the *Dai Mai*, the waist area is strong. Most important of all, the dantian is situated in this area. In order for qi to sink to the dantian, the waist area should be healthy and relaxed.

The main purpose of *Chung Mai* or the Thrusting Channel is to connect, communicate and mutually support the *Ren Mai*. This mutual support regulates qi in the kidneys, where original qi is produced. The channel also connects the spinal cord to the brain, nourishing the brain and therefore the spirit *(shen)*.

CHAPTER FOUR

Training Methods

Diligent practice of Chen Taijiquan will undoubtedly have a positive effect upon health. Taiji, like other movement arts or sports, can increase overall body strength, coordination and physical performance. Furthermore, it is a comprehensive martial system whose training curriculum reflects this point. Concentrated practice, over time, develops numerous aspects of an individual's character, promoting determination, perseverance and the correct application of intelligence. Many people begin Taiji searching for the health or martial benefits, but as awareness grows of its movement complexities, a deeper level of artistic or "spiritual" focus may develop. The multi-faceted nature of Taiji, at once a martial, medical, artistic and spiritual pursuit, lies behind its widespread appeal.

To achieve martial skill and enter the door to the deeper aspects of the art, a variety of training methods has evolved, including basic exercises, stance holding (*zhan zhuang*), single-posture training, *taolu* (form) training, power development exercises, weapons training and push hands drills for sensitivity. Past generations of masters assiduously analyzed and researched the various movements and skills through necessity. Prior to the invention of firearms, self and group preservation often relied upon both bare-hand and weaponry skills. There are no easy options if one seeks to develop higher-level abilities. While individual goals dictate the level of intensity during practice, combat efficiency necessitates a high degree of commitment in terms of time and effort. In the words of a well-known Chinese saying, the practitioner must be prepared to "eat bitterness" *(che ku)*.

Wuji Zhuang

"To train Taiji one must begin at Wuji; Yin and Yang, Open and Close, one must seek the truth."

This phrase provides the guideline for training. One must start from *wuji*, and then progress to Taiji. Without the foundation of the former, it is impossible to find the "real" Taiji. "Yin and Yang" is the core of Taiji, as the opposing yet combining elements of the two create Taiji. "Open and Close" *(Kai Her)* is a way of reconciling the differences, so that the two phases can harmonize. *"Yin and Yang, Open and Close"* denotes the essence of Taijiquan: the combination of motion and stillness, the coordination of internal and external, etc.

The implication of Taiji is to create opportunity from *wuji*. Although yin-yang is still not apparent, the opportunity for separation is still not apparent, but the potential for separation is already present. As soon as *wuji* stirs, Taiji occurs. From Taiji's "opening and closing," which means its continuously changing form, all things are possible. Taking the principle into Taijiquan, the door to Taiji begins with quiet standing—*wuji zhuang*.

Taijiquan is an internal martial art, requiring internal energy *(nei jing)* training as well as external physical training. The power and strength of internal energy are manifested in external actions. The internal force uses *jing*, *qi* and *shen* as foundation. When *jing* and qi are abundant, this can be manifested externally with muscles, tendons and bones into movements that are strong and forceful; pliable and flexible; fast as lightning; startling like thunder. The Taiji classics say: *"quan without gong, complete empty form"* and *"li is not as good as fa; fa is not as good as gong."*

To train internal skill, one must first train internal qi. This includes cultivation of qi, storage of qi and circulation of qi. Through prolonged training qi becomes fuller and stronger, filling the dantian, breaking through blockages in the *jingluo* (energy paths) and then saturating the whole body. The body is like an

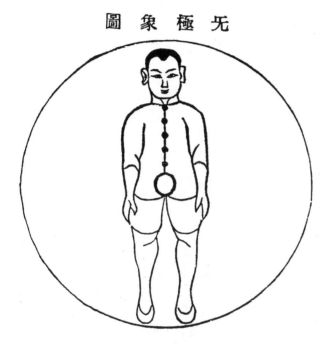

圖象極无

FIGURE 4.1
Chen Xin's illustration of "Wuji Zhuang"

無極者一物未有也太初以上渾渾
穆穆混混沌沌所謂大混沌者即此
時也學者上場打拳端然恭立合目
息氣兩手下垂身樁端正兩足並齊
心中一物無所著一念無所思穆穆
皇皇渾然如大混沌無極景象故其
形無可名名之曰無極象形也

inflated ball, full of elasticity and *peng jing*. With the silk-reeling movement of Chen Taijiquan, this energy can be circulated throughout the body.

The most basic method of training is *zhan zhuang*. *Zhan zhuang* is an exercise common to many Chinese martial arts, including Taijiquan. Usually the practitioner stands with arms held as if holding a large ball. However, the *zhan zhuang* exercise can be practiced using any of the end postures from the Taiji form. During "standing" practice a static posture is maintained for a period of time while using just enough strength to maintain the posture. To the casual observer it may appear as if little is happening; the experienced practitioner, though, is deeply absorbed in a variety of actions and sensations. Benefits of *zhan zhuang* include deep relaxation, strengthening of the legs and increased internal qi. The first requirement is to have a calm mind. This can be achieved in a number of ways—for instance, concentrating upon the Dantian, paying attention to one's breath, or silently counting.

Through standing practice, emphasis is placed upon developing awareness of and maintaining the most efficient and relaxed structural alignment necessary to hold the position. Prolonged practice, along with enhancing postural awareness and tranquillity of mind, greatly develops the strength of the legs. When the legs are strong and can bear weight firmly, then the upper body can relax and sink down into them, making the top more flexible. If the legs are not strong, the top is "afraid" of sinking down, and the body remains top-heavy and unrelaxed. The demands placed upon the legs are reflected in a traditional saying of Chenjiagou Village: *"Whoever drinks the water of Chenjiagou, their legs will shake."* Taijiquan requires lightness and sensitivity in the upper body. At the same time the lower body should have a feeling of extreme heaviness and connection to the ground. This feeling is often compared to a large tree with deep roots. While the branches move and sway in the wind, the trunk is solidly anchored by its roots.

The principles followed during *zhan zhuang* are carried over to the Taiji form, i.e., head erect, shoulders relaxed, elbows sunk down, chest relaxed, hips sunk, knees bent, etc. To correctly follow these basic requirements, though seemingly simple, requires intense concentration. As one develops competence in the different aspects during standing, the feelings and sensations that arise can be transferred to the Taiji form and push hands.

Standing Pole practice provides a means of increasing internal feeling and the circulation of qi. Regular standing for extended periods of time gives rise to acute body awareness as the practitioner learns to relax and sink their qi. By reducing the level of external stimulation, one can focus more closely upon sensations within the body. While the external body is still, internally the breath, blood and qi are circulating. This represents a state of balance, or "motion in stillness."

Practicing *zhan zhuang* has the following requirements: the top of the head should be held as though suspended lightly from above, or as if a light object were being supported on top of the head. If the head is not held steady, the object may fall. Hearing should be focused upon a point behind the head. The chin tucks in slightly so that the *Baihui* point (crown of the head) forms a line with the *Huiyin* point (between the sexual organs and the anus). If these requirements are followed, one will feel the qi sinking to the center and, at this point, the mind should be very calm.

A common problem in Standing Pole practice is holding the dantian too tightly. This causes an obstruction and prevents the qi from sinking down. If the qi is prevented from going to the dantian it rises to the chest, causing a feeling of tightness or oppression and adding to the workload of the heart. To ensure that the dantian remains relaxed, it is important that the musculature surrounding it plays little part in maintaining the body's position during standing.

Practicing the standing posture before the Taiji form helps to release tension from the body and mind, allowing higher-quality practice. The time spent on the *zhan zhuang* exercise should be increased slowly, starting with several minutes. During the first five to ten minutes, it is common to feel discomfort in certain parts of the body as you become aware of blockages of qi. At this stage it is important to persevere. For optimum benefits, the duration should be at least twenty, and preferably forty minutes.

Chan Ssu Gong (Silk-reeling Exercise)

Chan ssu gong is the method by which the silk-reeling force (*chan ssu jing*) of Chen Taijiquan is cultivated. *Chan ssu jing* should be present throughout all Taijiquan movement. As one becomes more knowledgeable about the subtle requirements of Chen Taijiquan, it is easy to become frustrated. It is particularly difficult for less-experienced students to practice the form while simultaneously being aware of the finer details of *chan ssu jing* movement, such as how to correctly shift weight; how to sink and relax; and how to turn the Dantian. To overcome this, silk-reeling energy skills are developed by continuously repeating small sections of movement. This makes it easier to concentrate on the deeper requirements, rather than on what comes next when practicing the whole form.

Silk-reeling exercises involve the uninterrupted practice of a single movement in a smooth, flowing manner. For the silk-reeling exercise to be effective, practice must be natural and relaxed. Awareness must be focused upon the movement of the hand, naturally adjusting to the movement of the body until there is a total coordination. Following the principle *"once any part is in motion, nothing remains still,"* the hands and legs co-operate harmoniously, while the torso turns freely without break. At this point the internal energy can be circulated freely, as any blockages in qi flow are smoothed out. Throughout the practice of silk-reeling, the mind leads all actions, directing strength through the joints in the correct order.

Each circle of the hands consists of two aspects—*shun-chan* and *ni-chan*. During *ni-chan* movements, one feels as if energy is being pushed out to the extremities. *Shun-chan* sees its return to the dantian. The *shun-chan* and *ni-chan* concepts refer not only to the movements of the hands, but to the folding of the chest and abdomen. Without this folding, the twining movements of the limbs cannot be expressed. Opening movements of the chest and abdomen are *ni-chan*, and closing movements are *shun-chan*. Without using force, these sensations must be cultivated if the full benefits of the silk-reeling exercises are to be attained. Concentrating upon the spiral movement of the arms rather than the coordination of the whole body misses the essence of silk-reeling training.

In martial terms, silk-reeling practice leads to an acute awareness of the body's center and how to maintain its equilibrium. Particular emphasis should be placed upon preserving the central equilibrium when changing

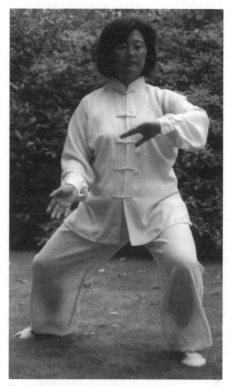

FIGURE 4.2 Davidine Sim practicing double-hand silk reeling.

the energy from *shun-chan* to *ni-chan*. Most people react to being pushed by stiffening up and losing the connection between body and center. The qi becomes blocked and balance is compromised as the center of gravity is lost. Good balance is a reflection of the level of silk-reeling energy present within the body. It is also a prerequisite for combative proficiency. Through mastering balance the practitioner can easily take advantage of, or deliberately cause, a weakness in an opponent's posture, while simultaneously preserving one's own center.

Silk-reeling exercises allow the practitioner to realize the unique twining movement method of Chen Taijiquan. The whole body spirals and twines simultaneously. Feng Ziqiang likens the upper body to a knot, while the legs are like screws twisting into the earth. With the development of silk-reeling energy throughout the body, the practitioner can transform the motion of an incoming force into a spiral motion. In this way force acting on the body can be smoothly neutralized during push hands exercises or in actual combat.

Ultimately, the practitioner seeks to unite the body into one functional unit. Chen Xiaowang suggests that failing to train in reeling silk can limit one to less than half the body's potential in any particular movement. To enable all the body's energy to come out when performing *fajing*, all of the body must be involved during the movement. Repeatedly training sets of single movements leads to an understanding of how the spiralling action of the waist initiates spiralling of the shoulder, elbow and wrist as well as the hips, knees and ankles.

Taolu (Forms)

Forms training is demanding. It requires the complete attention and participation of mind and body. Elements such as patience, persistence, *yi* (mind intent), strength, relaxation, and qi are essential in developing one's Taijiquan skills. Chen Zhaokui viewed the handform as the foundation upon which all the other skills of Taijiquan are built. Practicing the Taiji form is not simply a matter of mindlessly repeating the sequences. Each routine has been carefully researched and meticulously arranged. The forms are the culmination of practical experience, every posture and maneuver having been tried and tested then assembled to create the forms or routines we now know.

Great attention was given to the characteristics of the movements (whether hard or soft, difficult or easy, etc.) so that the complexities of the art could be learned progressively over time. For example, the beginning movements of the *Laojia* form are comparatively simple. The movements are comfortable and natural, with silk-reeling as the main principle. More softness and less hard movement make learning and practicing easier. Within the second routine, *Paocui*, the level of difficulty is greater. Movements are more complicated, faster and tighter, with shaking energy as the main principle. Through practice of the form comes an understanding of the various requirements of each movement—for instance, the positioning of hands and feet, bodily coordination through the movement, and how to position the body most advantageously for attack or defense.

While *zhan zhuang* is a fixed-position martial skill, practicing the form is a moving-posture skill. Taijiquan therefore is made up of *wuji zhuang* and *taiji zhuang*. In movement, the aim is to maintain firm rooting, while easily and naturally expressing the substantial and insubstantial through each change of direction or position.

Repetitive practice of the form leads to familiarity with the movements. In time coordination and flexibility are acquired throughout every move within the form. The quality of movement must be fluid and unpredictable, shifting instantaneously from slow to fast, from soft to hard, and from light to heavy. In his treatise on fighting methods, *Training for Sparring*, Chen Zhaokui writes:

> Emphasis on slow movements alone leads to slow strikes
> which an opponent can counter easily. Emphasis on fast moves
> only makes it difficult to feel the path of your energy
> and makes it easy to strike along a longer path than necessary.
> Being fast refers to the speed generated through familiarity
> of the energy path. It is a speed without loss of quality.

A feature recognized as unique to Chen Taijiquan is the use of both fast and slow movement. Within the Taijiquan classics is a saying that one should *"direct strength like reeling of silk from a cocoon"* and *"release strength like shooting an arrow."* Slow movements are characterized by alertness, and fast movements by control. This being said, the fast and slow within the Taijiquan form refer not only to the external form, but to how the inside movement manifests itself.

Consequently, fast and slow movement should arise naturally, without the feeling that a particular movement must be performed quickly or slowly. Feng Ziqiang suggests, *"The standard for determining quick or slow should be the unison of* yi, qi, shen *and* xing *[shape or body form]."*

While modern shortened versions of Chen Taijiquan are practiced as an introduction to the system, the main curriculum emphasizes two primary barehand routines. The first and more commonly practiced is the *Yi Lu* (First Route), the second being the more dynamic Cannon Fist or *Paocui* routine.

In comparison to the Cannon Fist, the movements of the first routine are relatively simple, with more emphasis placed upon softness *(rou)* than firmness *(gang)*. *Yi Lu* focuses upon the development of *chan ssu jing* through the twining and coiling movements of the limbs and body, interspersed with *fajing* (issuing energy) movements. In appearance, the form is relaxed, steady and stable, the limbs guided by the body in an unbroken sequence of opening and closing movements.

In practice, emphasis is placed upon slowness. Within each individual form, one begins slowly, executes the transition movements smoothly, and gradually settles into the final posture. Slowness is exhibited throughout each form, emphasizing each opening and closing, stretch and withdrawal, and up-and-down movement. Over a period of time, slow practice enables postures to be developed exactly, to fulfill the usage and application contained within. Each form teaches where the body position should be through each point of the technique, and slowness allows the body to become fixed in its postures. In this way, when it is speeded up the movement becomes natural and will not deviate. Posture and movement developed in this manner will become habitual and be useful not just when speeding up the movements of the form, but in pushing hands and *san shou* (free sparring).

To most other martial arts, the training of direct force and greater speed is seen as the natural means by which an opponent can be overcome. From this perspective, Taijiquan appears to conflict with nature. It seems that strength is naturally superior to weakness and speed more effective than slowness. Taijiquan philosophy, however, requires one to reverse this way of thinking. The practitioner must have confidence in the notion that a lesser strength can overcome a greater strength and that slowness can overcome speed. Speeding up movements before the postures have become fixed and exact leads only to a loss of detail and effectiveness. Therefore, the use of slowness represents one of the unique training methods of Taijiquan rather than its goal.

Calmness of the mind is essential in order to maintain the many details contained within the forms. Impatience can only lead to haste and a loss of detail. Calmness of mind enables qi to become quiet and then to follow the intention. In this way the intention can be developed, ensuring that the link between *shen* and qi is unbroken. This manner of practice eventually allows the practitioner of Taijiquan to execute whole-body movement throughout the form, unifying internal spirit or consciousness with the external form, thereby unite body and mind. Practicing slowly allows one to cultivate qi, increasing the health and vigor of the body. This provides the foundation from which martial stamina and skill can flourish.

In order not to hinder qi development, the forms should be practiced according to the principles, and one should not place a limit on each movement by focusing on one particular application. Every movement can have many possible applications. Considering each as part of a circle, one realizes that all points on the circle can represent a particular application, depending on the situation.

This use of coiling and twining movement of chan ssu jing is one of the defining characteristics of Chen style Taijiquan. Correct practice of the form using this method leads the student along the path to developing more effective *fajing* and, in time, to understanding how to apply and escape from *qinna* (joint-locking) movements. Diligent practice of the first form lays a strong foundation upon which more advanced skills can subsequently be built.

If one's reason for doing Taijiquan is its health benefits, then the first routine is sufficient. However, if the student seeks to develop martial effectiveness in addition to good health, the second routine should also be learned. As mentioned, the second form, Cannon Fist, is characterized by more complex movements with greater emphasis upon firmness rather than softness. It is performed at a much faster tempo than the first routine. Footwork is less fixed, as the routine contains many vigorous leaping, dodging and stamping movements. Where the first sequence seeks to develop the body's internal energy and stability through the use of silk-reeling, the Cannon Fist aims to prepare the practitioner for free fighting. Training the form requires the use of great bursts of energy. Unlike the *Yi Lu,* where applications can usually be understood in terms of a single opponent, the second form presupposes multiple opponents. The combat techniques express numerous *fajing,* speed, sweeps, elbow and shoulder techniques and sudden changes of attack and defense. Traditional wisdom suggests that one's

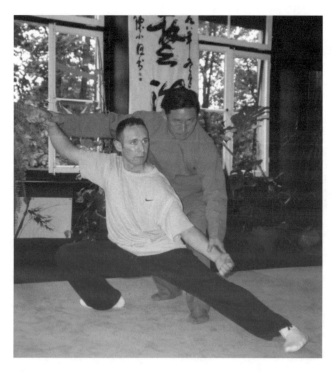

FIGURE 4.3
David Gaffney in posture "Dragon on the Ground," watched by Chen Xiaowang

training is not complete until both routines have been mastered. Diligent practice of the first routine is seen as vital to develop the internal energy. Subsequent training in the Cannon Fist form consolidates and expresses this energy.

Taijiquan is a complex and practical martial art. Its efficient use rests upon an understanding of its underlying principles if one is to realize the inner content and avoid the practice of pretty but empty "flowery fists." Chen Zhaokui emphasized the need to always seek to bring out the most difficult, the most demanding and the most detailed aspects of the movements within the form. At no time should the practitioner cheat to get around a demanding movement. For example, one takes a low stance during the Dragon on the Ground *(Que Di Long)* posture, and then, even more difficult, changes to the next position through arced movement.

Fundamental to the correct practice of Taijiquan is the constant involvement of the *yi*, or mind, all movements within the form arising from the mind's "intent." The *yi* moves the qi, which in turn moves the body. Training the Taiji form requires the practitioner to develop a deep level of concentration upon the internal sensations of the body, at all times focusing upon the precise movement being performed. In terms of strictness and attention to detail, even the smallest detail must be clearly executed, with no brushing over a movement that is unclear. Each movement within the sequence should be carefully considered as to its function and characteristics—whether it is relaxed enough; where to open and close; whether to turn in the foot; if there is enough spiral movement, etc. The practitioner meticulously works out the requirements, slowly reducing the number of shortcomings and faults. With this mindset each repetition of the form should lead to new discoveries and understandings, and ultimately mastery.

To develop a deep level of *yi* and qi, the form must be practiced correctly for a period of time. Distinct stages must be passed through. First the sequence must be mastered until it becomes very familiar. At this stage emphasis is placed primarily upon attaining looseness in the joints and correct body structure. Initially, training should center on standardizing the movements of the form as closely as possible to fulfill the body requirements of Chen Taijiquan. Each time the student comes to a fixed posture—for example, Lazily Tying Coat *(Lan Zha Yi)*, Single Whip *(Dan Bian)* or Preparing Form *(Taiji Qi Shi)*—he or she should focus strictly upon each part of the body, making sure that it conforms to the principles. This process requires considerable mental effort if the student is to avoid deviating from the correct path. Though many people can quote the requirements of Taijiquan and verses from the Taijiquan classics, real understanding can only come through training these into one's body. For instance, it is not enough to know that the shoulders must be relaxed *(song jien)*; the practitioner must experiment to discover how to relax them and to what degree. Or when containing or storing the chest *(han xiong)*, how is this achieved? At what point is it sufficiently stored? Too much and the waist collapses, too little and the shoulder tightens.

Chen Zhaokui lists sixteen requirements that must be present throughout each posture:

- Eye movement (the direction of the eyes)
- The shape of the hands, and how the hand changes as the movement is being performed
- *Shun-chan* and *ni-chan* (silk-reeling) of the arms
- Footwork (how to execute changes when stepping)
- *Shun-chan* and *ni-chan* of the legs
- Opening and closing of the chest and back
- Rising and falling of the buttocks
- Dantian rotation (waist and lower abdomen)
- Shifting weight (the relationship of substantial and insubstantial)
- Beginning and end points, as well as the transition movements of the upper and lower limbs
- How much strength to use, and where the strength should be concentrated (i.e., where is the attack point?)
- Position and direction of posture

- The rise and fall of spiral movement (top and bottom coordination)
- The change in tempo (alternating slow and fast)
- Breathing (coordination of breathing and movement)
- Listening

The requirements are not rigid measurements but must be experienced and refined through constant practice. Their subtlety is reflected in an ancient Taijiquan saying: *"Only the gods know, impossible to transmit orally."* To the beginning student, the body requirements of Chen Taijiquan sometimes seem almost impossibly strict. However, by going through this process, higher levels of skill can be reached in a step-by-step manner. As one becomes aware of how to keep the mind clear and calm, and how to sink qi to the dantian, these feelings can be focused upon and strengthened during the fixed postures.

Once the form can be performed naturally, the internal energy can develop. With each completed posture, the qi sinks to the dantian and from there is distributed throughout the body.

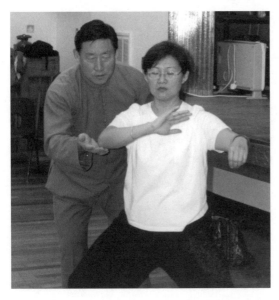

FIGURE 4.4
Chen Xiaowang showing movement principle to Davidine Sim

Through continual, diligent practice more qi is accumulated and stored in the dantian. Chen Zhenglei likens the dantian to a large river, saying that if the water level is not sufficiently high, then water cannot flow to the smaller tributaries downstream. So, if the dantian has not filled with qi, qi cannot be pushed out to the extremities.

When the fixed postures have been standardized and the basic requirements fulfilled, the practitioner then must consider the movement principles—for example, using the waist as the axis, moving sectionally, etc. At this stage, one must seek the correct route of each movement in the form, incorporating the basic requirements and movement principles. As these are realized, the internal energy from the dantian can be accurately directed to the appropriate point, depending upon which movement is being performed.

Following the development of basic skills, the form is a training method to prepare the body for combat and practical usage of the skills. In an essay entitled "Training Method of Chen Taiji Routine and Push Hands," Chen Zhaokui writes:

> Every position should be precise and each destination
> [intention] should be clear. You should know the opponent's
> position. Then it will involve your hand, body, footwork,
> sight and hearing.

Every movement and every step within the form is training for a particular purpose, and importance should be placed equally on all of them, not just those with obvious martial applications. Over time, conscientious practice and study of the form allow the practitioner to identify and develop both the attacking and defensive facets of the art.

Hong Junsheng, a senior student of Chen Fa-ke, said that in terms of combat, Taijiquan requires the neutralization of an incoming force through rotational movement to "lead the attacker off harmlessly" (yin jin luo kong). Whichever part of the body is attacked, that part turns in the same direction as the attacking force to neutralize its effect. At the same time, the body continues to rotate to naturally form a circle that is made up of, on the one side, soft neutralizing energy and on the other, hard issuing energy.

From a defensive standpoint, the aim is to gain the ability to entice an opponent into emptiness. This requires training to a level where one can stick, connect, adhere and follow, neither losing contact with nor resisting the opponent. Offensive *gong fu* is acquired through the cultivation of the eight energy methods *(ba fa)* of *peng, lu, ji, an, cai, lie, zhou* and *kao*. It is said that with the development of the Taijiquan skills, a level of ability is eventually reached *"where four ounces can overcome a thousand pounds."*

To reach this stage, the form must be practiced until it becomes continuous, with one movement flowing naturally into the next, outwardly relaxed but inwardly strong. Where hard and soft elements are combined, the upper and lower body are co-ordinated, and the internal and external *(yi* and *li)* work closely together. Movement is refined, and all stiff, clumsy and uneven actions are eliminated.

Practice must strictly adhere to the rules of Taijiquan if one is to reach a high level of proficiency. The number of forms practiced and the degree of athletic difficulty should take into account the relative strength or weakness, age and health of the practitioner. For less-experienced students, it is preferable that movements be large, comfortable and open. The expression of roundness, fullness and continuous motion, as well as the alternation of opening and closing movements, can be more clearly seen when the spiralling silk-reeling circles are larger.

Whether the form is practiced in a high or low stance is decided according to personal preference. In the early stages of training, low postures allow one to develop the foundation strength of the lower body, as well as to more clearly see the folding movements of the waist and turning of the legs. As the level of skill increases it is normal for the postures to become higher. This higher stance is, however, extremely agile, the practitioner being able to change naturally and easily between high and low positions. For the older beginner, a higher position may be more comfortable. Above all, in practicing the form one should let naturalness be the guiding principle.

The pace of development cannot be forced. Paradoxically, the more you try to hurry, the more difficult it is to reach achievement. Chen Fa-ke illustrated this point with a story about two prospective students who wished to learn from him. The first had considerable martial art experience, which he was quick to make known. After questioning the master as to how long it would take to achieve a high level of skill, Chen Fa-ke replied, "In three years expect small success, in five years expect medium success, and in ten years great success." Upon hearing this, the student immediately boasted that he would train one hundred times harder than his fellow students and would achieve mastery in one year.

In contrast, the second student modestly requested to learn from the master, endeavoring to do his best and to practice for as long as his teacher felt necessary. Comparing the two students, Chen Fa-ke remarked that the impatience of the first student would hinder his progress, as he was full of his past experience and his mind was not calm. The second student, on the other hand, could look forward to greater success, as his mind was open and he was in no hurry.

Chen style Taijiquan can be divided into two frames today: Old and New (*Laojia* and *Xinjia*, respectively), each consisting of a First Routine and Cannon Fist. From the time of Chen Changxing (1771-1853), the Taijiquan exponents of Chenjiagou Village practiced the *Laojia* routines. A synthesis of the five routines passed down from Chen Taijiquan creator Chen Wangting, the *Laojia Yi Lu* (First Route) and *Er Lu* (Second Route/Cannon Fist) preserved many of the movements and all of the movement principles of the older routines. The *Laojia Yi Lu* consists of seventy-four postures, usually taking approximately ten minutes to complete.

The hand form provides the blueprint for developing the martial skills of Chen Taijiquan. A complex training tool, it incorporates many elements which, when combined, enable the practitioner to fully develop fighting skills. Chen Xin's book, *Illustrated*

Explanation of Chen Family Taijiquan, sometimes referred to as the Bible of Chen Taiji, provides a detailed breakdown of the Old Frame first series form and the purpose of its various movements, dividing the form into thirteen distinct sections.

Chen Family Taijiquan Boxing: *Laojia Yi Lu* (First Routine—74 Postures)

Section One

1. Preparing Form *(Taiji Qi Shi)*

2. Buddha's Warrior Attendant Pounds Mortar *(Jin Gang Dao Dui)*

In the first section, the Taiji yin-yang philosophy is clearly expressed. The opening form begins with *wuji* stance. Following the principles of Daoism, from stillness comes movement. With the beginning of movement, Taiji is created with its constituent parts of yin and yang. This is reflected in the alternation of soft and hard, empty and full, etc. In his *Treatise on Taijiquan*, eighteenth-century Taijiquan master Wang Zongyue wrote, "Taiji is born in wuji, the incorporation of stillness and movement, the mother of Yin and Yang."

Section Two

3. Lazily Tying Coat *(Lan Zha Yi)*

4. Six Sealing and Four Closing *(Liu Feng Si Bi)*

5. Single Whip *(Dan Bian)*

6. Buddha's Warrior Attendant Pounds Mortar *(Jin Gang Dao Dui)*

Section two further expands upon Taiji yin-yang theory. When

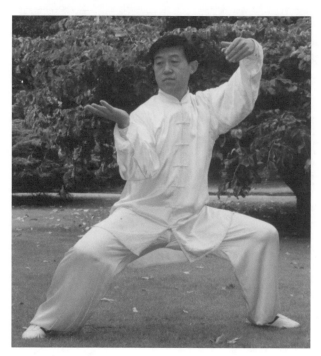

FIGURE 4.5
Chen Zhenglei in
'Six Sealing and Four
Closing'

still, yin and yang combine to form a whole. When in motion, they separate, producing the two forms or *Liang Yi.*

Section Three

7. White Crane Spreads Its Wings *(Bai He Liang Che)*

8. Walking Obliquely *(Xie Xing)*

9. Brushing Knees *(Lou Xi)*

These postures clearly illustrate the transition from *Liang Yi* to *Si Xiang*. In philosophical terms, the two *(Liang Yi)* become four *(Si Xiang)*. The four main directions of *kan, li, zhen* and *dui* are expressed.

Section Four

10. Stepping Three Steps *(Shan San Bu)*

11. Walking Obliquely *(Xie Xing)*

During the fourth section *Si Xiang* becomes *Bagua*. In other words, the four further subdivide into the eight. In philosophical terms, the eight trigrams of *Kan, Li, Zhen, Dui, Qian, Kun, Gen* and *Sun* provide symbolic representation of the eight basic methods of Taijiquan: warding off, diverting, squeezing, pressing down, plucking, splitting, elbowing, and bumping.

Section Five:

12. Brushing Knees *(Lou Xi)*

13. Stepping Three Steps *(Shan San Bu)*

14. Hidden Thrust Punch and Whirling Upper Arms *(Yan Shou Hong Quan)*

15. Buddha's Warrior Attendant Pounds Mortar *(Jin Gang Dao Dui)*

Here emphasis is on accumulating as well as expending *jing* and then returning to the original Taiji posture. *Wuji* is paramount. When practicing Taijiquan, every movement begins with *wuji*, becomes Taiji, and then returns to wuji.

Section Six

16. Flinging Body *(Pie Sen Quan)*

17. Green Dragon Out of the Water *(Qing Lung Chu Shui)*

18. Double Pushing Hands *(Shuang Tui Shou)*

19. Fist Beneath Elbow *(Zhou Di Kan Quan)*

20. Step Back and Whirl Arms *(Dao Juan Hong)*

21. White Crane Spreads Its Wings *(Bai He Liang Che)*

22. Walking Obliquely *(Xie Xing)*

This section covers a number of important training methods—for instance, turning the body, leaning, folding the body and stepping backwards.

Section Seven

23. Flash with Back *(Shan Tong Bei)*

24. Hidden Thrust Punch and Whirling Upper Arms *(Yan Shou Hong Quan)*

25. Six Sealing and Four Closing *(Liu Feng Si Bi)*

26. Single Whip *(Dan Bian)*

Section seven helps the practitioner develop the ability to turn their body freely in response to an opponent's action, remaining balanced and stable throughout. When one moves with agility, an opponent's incoming force can be led to emptiness.

Section Eight

27. Cloud Hands *(Yun Shou)*

28. High Pat on Horse *(Gao Tan Ma)*

29. Brushing the Right Foot *(You Pai Jiao)*

30. Brushing the Left Foot *(Zuo Pai Jiao)*

31. Kick with the Left Heel *(Zuo Deng Gen)*

32. Forward Twist Step *(Qian Zang Ao Bu)*

33. Punch the Ground *(Zhi Di Chui)*

34. Double Raise Kick *(Ti Er Qi)*

35. Protecting the Heart *(Hu Xing Quan)*

36. Tornado Foot *(Xuan Feng Jiao)*

37. Kick with the Right Heel *(You Deng Gen)*

38. Hidden Thrust Punch and Whirling Upper Arms
    (Yan Shou Hong Quan)

39. Small Catch and Hit *(Xiao Qin Da)*

40. Embrace Head and Push Mountain *(Bao Toh Tui Shan)*

41. Six Sealing and Four Closing *(Liu Feng Si Bi)*

42. Single Whip *(Dan Bian)*

This section develops a diverse range of attacking and defending methods. Several movements work on developing the *bufa* or footwork skills of Chen Taijiquan. For instance, Cloud Hands trains the sidestepping method and Small Catch and Hit trains the ability to enter an opponent's space stealthily.

A number of postures focus specifically on attacking techniques with the legs. The Left and Right Heel Kicks allow the practitioner to attack with the feet. Double Raise Kick adds the extra dimension of leaping into the air, while Tornado Foot teaches how to kick while turning the body in a complete circle, maintaining balance throughout.

Embrace Head and Push Mountain emphasizes closing one's body internally; Single Whip enhances the coordination of the upper and lower body; and Protecting the Heart allows the practitioner to protect his head, heart and knee.

The sixteen postures of section eight are geared towards meeting a group attack, and the sequence should be performed as if it were a single posture. Each technique is executed without pause, and all actions are well co-ordinated. Considering the most useful tactics when fighting, Chen Zhaokui suggested that the priority must be to wipe out the enemy, with preserving oneself being secondary.

Section Nine

43. Forward Trick *(Qian Zhao)*

44. Backward Trick *(Hou Zhao)*

45. Parting the Wild Horse's Mane *(Ye Ma Feng Zhong)*

46. Six Sealing and Four Closing *(Liu Feng Si Bi)*

47. Single Whip *(Dan Bian)*

48. Jade Girl Works Shuttles *(Yu Nu Quan Shuo)*

49. Lazily Tying Coat *(Lan Zha Yi)*

50. Six Sealing and Four Closing *(Liu Feng Si Bi)*

51. Single Whip *(Dan Bian)*

The postures of section nine develop the *Jiao Shou* or "Engaging Hand" tactics. Each posture is an attacking movement until qi returns to the dantian with the Single Whip. During Forward and Backward Trick, the practitioner strikes to the left and right sides training the hand and eye methods; Parting the Wild Horse's Mane is a swift entry method "splitting" *(lie)* an opponent's body. "Jade Girl Works Shuttles" is characterized by turning the body and then directly entering the opponent's space. Chen Changxing, in his *Important Words on Martial Applications*, wrote:

> Heart must take the lead,
> intention must conquer the opponent,
> body must attack him,
> steps must pass through him.

Section Ten

52. Cloud Hands *(Yun Shou)*

53. Shake Foot and Stretch Down *(Bai Jiao Die Cha)*

54. Golden Rooster Stands on One Leg *(Jin Ji Du Li)*

55. Step Back and Whirl Arms *(Dao Juan Hong)*

56. White Crane Spreads Its Wings *(Bai He Liang Chi)*

57. Walking Obliquely *(Xie Xing)*

58. Flash with Back *(Shan Tong Bei)*

59. Hidden Thrust Punch and Whirling Upper Arms *(Yan Shou Hong Quan)*

60. Six Sealing and Four Closing *(Liu Feng Si Bi)*

61. Single Whip *(Dan Bian)*

The postures of this section should be *"executed in one breath,"* without being separated. So again, this sequence should be approached as if it were one posture made up of a number of smaller postures. The Shake Foot and Stretch Down posture helps to develop Taijiquan's crescent kicking method (where the leg circles out from the body in an arc). When stretching down, lower body strength and flexibility are enhanced. By practicing the movement in a low position with open hips and strong, firm legs, the upper body will become very loose and free. During the Golden Rooster Stands on One Leg posture, raising the knees in the transition movement Stamp Towards Heaven trains how to attack with the knees. All the other postures are repeated movements from previous sections.

Section Eleven

62. Cloud Hands *(Yun Shou)*

63. High Pat on Horse *(Gao Tan Ma)*

64. Crossed Foot Kick *(Shi Zhi Jiao)*

65. Punch to Crotch *(Zhi Dang Chui)*

66. White Ape Presents Fruit *(Bai Yuan Xian Guo)*

67. Six Sealing and Four Closing *(Liu Feng Si Bi)*

68. Single Whip *(Dan Bian)*

Movements not performed previously include: Crossed Foot Kick, training the practitioner in the technique of leaning with the upper body *(kao)* before kicking; Punch to Crotch, a life-threatening technique once a high degree of ability in *fajing* has been developed; and White Ape Presents Fruit, a rapid upward entering movement.

Section Twelve

69. Stepping Forward with Seven Stars *(Shang Bu Qi Xing)*

70. Step Back to Ride the Tiger *(Xia Bu Kua Hu)*

During the first movement, the practitioner opens the right leg and sits back, storing energy in readiness to propel oneself forward; Stepping Forward with Seven Stars trains the method of advancing with a step; Step Back to Ride the Tiger facilitates the attainment of upper and lower body synchronization.

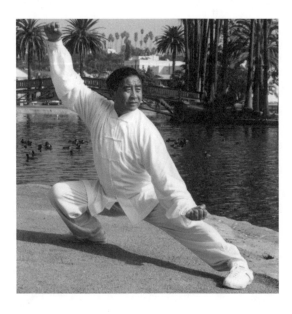

FIGURE 4.6
Zhu Tiancai in 'Step Forward with Seven Stars'

Section Thirteen

71. Turn Back and Wave Double Lotus *(Zhuan Shen Shuang Bai Lian)*

72. Head-on Blow *(Dang Tou Pao)*

73. Buddha's Warrior Attendant Pounds Mortar *(Jin Gang Dao Dui)*

74. Closing Form *(Taiji Shou Si)*

The final section trains the following skills: Turn Back and Wave Double Lotus allows one to practice two methods, one being how to turn the body, the other the combination of *shang peng, xia da* or upper *peng,* lower attack; the Head-on Blow is a means of protecting the face, head and heart.

Laojia's Cannon Fist *(Paocui)* routine is usually performed in a fast, explosive manner. From start to finish, the form takes only about four minutes to complete. Containing many vigorous movements such as leaping, stamping and dodging, the Cannon Fist is an important training method for readying one's body for actual combat. Traditionally this form was only taught after the student had reached a level of some proficiency in the first routine. Generally this would mean a minimum of about three years' consistent practice. Many modern practitioners are unwilling to spend long periods of time practicing basic exercises and the first routine. A failure to understand the underlying Taijiquan principles leads to the form being performed in an external manner lacking the characteristics of Taijiquan.

FIGURE 4.7
Chen Zhenglei demonstrating 'Paocui'

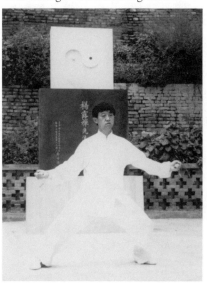

Chen Family Taijiquan Boxing: *Laojia Paocui* (Cannon Fist—43 Postures)

1. Preparing Form *(Taiji Qi Shi)*

2. Buddha's Warrior Attendant Pounds Mortar *(Jin Gang Dao Dui)*

3. Lazily Tying Coat *(Lan Zha Yi)*

4. Six Sealing and Four Closing *(Liu Feng Si Bi)*

5. Single Whip *(Dan Bian)*

6. Protecting the Heart *(Hu Xing Quan)*

7. Walk Obliquely *(Xie Xing)*

8. Buddha's Warrior Attendant Pounds Mortar *(Jin Gang Dao Dui)*

9. Flinging Body *(Pie Sen Quan)*

10. Punch to Crotch *(Zhi Dang Chui)*

11. Cutting Hands *(Zhan Shou)*

12. Turn Flowers Out and Brandish Sleeves *(Fan Shen Wu Xiu)*

13. Hidden Thrust Punch *(Yan Shou Hong Quan)*

14. Move and Hinder with Elbow *(Yao Lan Zhou)*

15. Big Cloud Hands and Small Cloud Hands *(Da Yun Shou Xiao Yun Shou)*

16. Jade Girl Works Shuttles *(Yu Nu Quan Shuo)*

17. Ride Animal in the Reverse Direction *(Dao Qi Lu)*

18. Hidden Thrust Punch *(Yan Shou Hong Quan)*

19. Wrap Crackers *(Guo Bian)*

20. Beast's Head Pose *(Shou Tou Shi)*

21. Splitting Pose *(Pia Jia Zi)*

22. Turn Flowers Out and Brandish Sleeves *(Fang Shen Wu Xiu)*

23. Hidden Thrust Punch *(Yan Shou Hong Quan)*

24. Tame Tiger *(Fu Hu)*

25. Rubbing Eyebrow Thrust *(Muo Mei Hong)*

26. Yellow Dragon Stirs Water Three Times *(Huang Long San Jiao Shui)*

27. Dash Leftward *(Zuo Chong)*

28. Dash Rightward *(You Chong)*

29. Hidden Thrust Punch *(Yan Shou Hong Quan)*

30. Sweeping Leg *(Shao Dang Tui)*

31. Hidden Thrust Punch *(Yan Shou Hong Quan)*

32. Linking Cannons *(Quan Pao Quan)*

33. Hidden Thrust Punch *(Yan Shou Hong Quan)*

34. Pound Crossed Wrists *(Dao Cha)*

35. Attack Twice with Left and Right Forearms *(Zuo You Erh Hong)*

36. Turning Head Cannon *(Hui Tou Dan Men Pao)*

37. Taiji Cannons *(Taiji Pao)*

38. Move and Hinder With Elbow *(Yao Lan Zhou)*

39. Smooth Elbow *(Shun Lan Zhou)*

40. The Cannon Out of the Bosom *(Wuo Di Pao)*

41. Go Straight into the Well *(Hui Tou Jing Lan Zhi Ru)*

42. Buddha's Warrior Attendant Pounds Mortar *(Jin Gang Dao Dui)*

43. Closing Form *(Taiji Shou Shi)*

After successfully defending himself numerous times from challenges by top martial arts masters of the day, seventeenth-generation master Chen Fa-ke re-evaluated the *Laojia* routines. He sought to discern how the routines could be changed to enhance the practitioner's ability with regard to the practical usage of the form. Chen Fa-ke subsequently developed the *Xinjia* (New Frame) forms by increasing the number of *qinna* and *fajing* movements.

The forms are not simply sequences of movements and techniques to be memorized and then repeated in a parrot-like fashion. Rather, they are training tools with which one can hone the ability to move and respond in a relaxed, natural and powerful way. Chen Xiaowang, in his article "The Fajing of Chen Style Taijiquan," suggests that an appropriate attitude when practicing the form is to train diligently, ignoring tiredness and accepting the need to work hard.

Stances and Stepping Method

"Cultivate the roots, and the branches and leaves will be abundant."

A primary point for the development of good Taijiquan is to nurture your root *(ken)* and create a strong foundation. "Root" in this sense means an unshakeable and steady lower plane *(xia pan)*. Eighteenth-generation Chen family master Chen Zhaopei stressed the importance of cultivating the lower body:

> If one cannot come to recognize how the weight moves
> distinctly backward and forward between the two legs,
> then the upper and lower cannot work together and connect.
> If the upper and lower cannot connect, then you cannot absorb
> the opponent's force, you cannot use his force.

In an article titled "Important Words on Martial Applications," fourteenth-generation master Chen Changxing emphasized the need to be aware of footwork and stepping strategies.

He wrote:

> Those wishing to advance the left must first enter right,
> those wishing to advance the right must first enter left;
> when taking a step, heel first touches the ground,
> ten toes should grasp the ground, steps should be steady,
> body should be serious and heavy...

The stances and stepping exercises of Chen Taijiquan are designed to build leg power and to develop basic footwork strategies. Often quoted in old Taijiquan classics is the saying that energy arises from the feet, is generated by the legs and is controlled by the waist. For the body to be steady the root must be firm. Footwork and stance training, therefore, represent one of the most fundamental building blocks of Taijiquan.

Whether in advance or defense, the foremost requirement is maintaining lower plane stability. This stability should be present in all maneuvers: *peng* (warding off); changing direction; dodging; jumping and leaping; kicking; stepping in, etc. A failure to understand this important point will hinder progress. *Xia pan gong* involves the lower body strength—using the feet as the base and legs as support, with the *dang* rounded, flexible and naturally sunken and stable.

No matter what *bufa* is being employed, the movement should contain both stillness and motion. Taiji classics say *"taking steps like a cat."* In other words, one's footwork must be stable yet nimble. Chen Xiaowang teaches that each time the Taijiquan practitioner takes a step, the feeling should be as if they were approaching a precipice or thin ice, the intention being to test the ground while in a position to rapidly withdraw if the environment is not favorable. Therefore, the weight must be stable on the supporting leg before lifting the other leg to make a step. When withdrawing, the step should be taken smoothly without balance becoming shaky or adjusting one's upper body. Stepping back has to be firm and stable. In the words of Chen Zhaokui: "Advancing requires lightness and softness, withdrawing requires firmness and steadiness."

The most commonly used stances are the *gung bu* (bow stance) and *xu bu* (empty stance). However, the system also incorporates *du li bu* (single leg stance), *pu bu* (crouching stance) and *zhou pan* (sitting stances). Of these, the *gung bu* is considered to be most important. Weight is distributed 60%–70% on the substantial leg, the remainder on the insubstantial leg. Both legs are opened with an opposite energy, feet placed slightly wider than the shoulders. The characteristic bow shape in the *gung bu* is formed by opening and relaxing the *kua* and rounding the crotch (*yuan dang*). Chen Taijiquan's requirements on the lower body are very precise. In developing the lower body stability one must practice opening the *dang*; rounding the *dang*; drawing in the *dang*; raising the *dang*— all executed with qi down to the dantian, weight bearing down and *jing* generated from the feet. Balance is firm and solid, and the practitioner can simultaneously attend to the front and back, and left and right directions.

The Taiji classics say that we must *"plant deep in order to grow roots."* For the lower plane to be strong, the hip joints have to sit down strongly. The buttocks line up with the heels. In order to allow the weight of the upper body to press down, the knee joints must be firm and strong. *Jing* in both feet feels as if it is driven into the ground below. The front supporting leg is solid and sunken into the ground, with the big toe holding in the weight. The back leg is also firmly planted, with the little toe holding in the weight. The center of gravity drops in between the legs. The movement of the waist and *dang* facilitates weight change. If these requirements are fulfilled, the stance has the structural strength of an arched bridge.

To maintain the hands and feet in the most effective application range, the practitioner must execute stepping moves competently. Failure to do so, with poor footwork, causes the body's center of gravity to become unbalanced once in motion. Each time the center is unbalanced it provides an opportunity for an opponent to attack. Consequently, the practitioner must work diligently to increase the versatility and changeability of their footwork, and not let their opponent take control. When stepping out one must choose the most advantageous position in which to place the foot. By using either *tau* (controlling the opponent's outside leg) or *qa* (controlling his inside space), the opponent's root can be upset.

Footwork and stance training teaches how to distinguish between emptiness and solidity and to differentiate where each should be. When moving, there is a clear distinction between which foot is substantial and which insubstantial *(xu shi fen ming)*. After a period of training, people learn how to change the center of gravity between the two legs. However, further training is necessary if they are to know how to effectively change their footwork.

The ability to change footwork is a prerequisite of various techniques of the upper body. There is a number of circumstances in which the footwork of the Taijiquan practitioner should be changed—in particular, when the current stance has reached the limit of its travel while maintaining all postural requirements. An example would be pushing with both arms fully extended, and the knee already bent so as to be directly above the toes. To maintain the forward movement, it is necessary to change the position of the feet. Changing steps can be performed either by advancing the forward foot approximately half a step, with the rear foot following up the same distance, or by the rear foot advancing and becoming the front foot.

Supplementary training for *xia pan gong* includes low horse stance; low bow stance; crouch stance; one-legged squats; *da-lu* push hands; and taking single postures from the *taolu* to practice *fajing*. The basic stance and footwork training cannot be omitted if high-level skills are to be attained. With persistent practice over time, one's lower plane strength will be established, with the ability to maintain balance under all circumstances. The importance of this is reflected in Chen Xin's saying *"that while the hand enters threefold, the leg enters sevenfold."*

Single-Posture Training

Once the concepts behind the Taijiquan forms and push hands methods have been understood and trained until they are very familiar, then practice can be taken a step further with the introduction of single-posture training. At this stage, the form is dismantled as selected movements are trained repeatedly. By taking out the most effective application and *fajing* movements, the practitioner can enhance combat requirements such as accuracy and speed. To develop martial ability, the methods of form, push hands and single-posture training must all be utilized. The three are closely interrelated: push hands is the means by which the accuracy of the form can be tested; form training is the foundation upon which effective push hands skills are built; single-posture training is the means by which martial skill is brought out. Chen Zhaokui stressed the importance of single-posture practice:

> Some applications of the movement cannot be used
> in push hands. For example elbow strikes, leg methods
> and also attacking vital points of an opponent, or qinna.
> Also some very fast *fajing* movements in the form
> cannot be done successively, as it would be too exhausting.

To many, the single-posture training appears boring and monotonous. However, repeating individual movements numerous times greatly develops the ability to use them practically. Much single-posture practice centers on the development of effective *fajing* skills. Nevertheless, there must be no deviation from the core principles of Taijiquan. Every time force is emitted, the movement should be loose, pliable and elastic, rather than rigid and stiff. Even when performing very fast and powerful actions, the practitioner should seek the silk-reeling spiral path and not straight-line movement. The whole body is involved, and there is a clear distinction between the storing and releasing of energy.

Single-movement practice can be divided into several categories, starting with those movements executed while stationary. Examples include the stamping action at the end of Buddha's Warrior Attendant Pounds Mortar *(Jin Gang Dao Dui)*, The Hidden Thrust Punch *(Yan Shou Hong Quan)* and the Green Dragon Out of the Water *(Qing Lung Chu Shui)*. Additional single move-

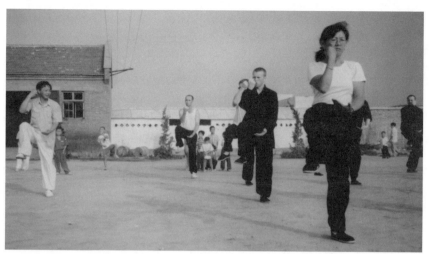

FIGURE 4.8 Gou Kongjie leading a training session in Zhenghou, China.

ments include those that involve stepping, for example, stepping forward using *fajing* while practicing the energy methods of Taijiquan (e.g. *cai, lie, zhou, kao*), and retreating movements, as in the posture Step Back and Whirl Arms *(Dao Juan Hong)*.

Fajing

Defense and attack are features common to all martial arts. Generally, defense is seen as *rou* (soft), attack as *gang* (hard). A unique feature of Chen style Taijiquan is the frequent use of *fajing* or the explosive issuing of energy by any part of the body. Along with the fist, elbow, shoulder, knee and foot used in the external martial arts, Chen Taijiquan requires the practitioner to be able to *fajing* with whichever part comes into contact with an opponent. This can be used to throw or strike an opponent. Following the principle of yin and yang, Taijiquan combines the hard and soft energies smoothly and interchangeably. Not only can any part of the body *fajing*, but strength can be changed internally, blending attack into defense and vice versa.

The key to effectively releasing force lies in relaxing the body and mind and using the waist. To emit energy, the ultimate aim in Chen Taijiquan, is to harness one hundred percent of the body's strength during a movement. To do this the energy from the feet is generated through the legs to the waist, where it is intensified by the spiral movement, then joined with the energy produced in the arm and fist. *Jing* or internal strength must start from both feet. If not applied from a firmly rooted position then no source of power is available. Without resistance from the floor, energy cannot go through the body sectionally to form a complete system. Without the rebounding energy from the ground, powerful whole-body strength cannot be activated.

The first requirement in *fajing* is letting the body relax (*fangsong*) in order to gather energy and let qi sink down to the feet. Then with a quick turn of the waist, with the energy generated from the ground through the feet, the internal strength is discharged. From the dantian it divides into two—half goes out to the hands and the other half goes down to the feet. For example, during the movement Hidden Thrust Punch (*Yang Shou Hong Quan*), after storing energy, the waist turns to the left, and the body's energy, following the turning of the waist, is emitted through the back, shoulder, arm and right fist. This is the movement's upward energy.

Fajing, like all the other actions of Chen Taijiquan, follows the *chan ssu jing* principle. Spiralling energy begins in the kidney area of the waist, goes down to the feet, and then rebounds to whichever part is going to express one's power. It is said that the well-trained Taijiquan exponent should be able to use any part of their body to release energy. So when power is being emitted it is not limited to the hands; it could be in your shoulder, your back, your elbow, your knee, your hip, etc.

Before *fajing*, energy must be stored by allowing the qi to sink and collect fully in the dantian. Releasing energy before this point will result in a movement powered largely by the upper body. Immediately relaxing after the *fajing* causes the body to recoil, collecting the energy in readiness for the next movement.

Paradoxically, the more softness that can be utilized during the storing phase, the more hardness can be achieved on release. Beginning students are often too anxious to use *fajing* when practicing their Taijiquan forms. At this stage, *fangsong* or relaxation and looseness is most important. Having acquired the ability to *fangsong*, one is then ready to correctly train oneself to do *fajing*. During the *fangsong* process, all stiff energy within the body is gradually released. The body must be totally relaxed and rid of all stiff energy in order to send all the power out rather than retaining it in the arms and body. Only when the entire body is relaxed and not one bit of stiff energy remains can force be completely emitted from the body.

When emitting energy, the movement must be unforced. Forcing the movement increases the stiffness and resistance of the body. Correct execution of *fajing* should be undetectable by an opponent before release. Speed and power are greatly increased by reducing the level of energy released en route to the end point. Any tension within the muscle (or joints that have not been fully opened) will provide resistive forces that pull the striking area back. This causes energy to be released through the trajectory of the motion, lessening the amount of energy getting through to the end point. Tension should only be manifested at the end point, that is, the point of impact. The moment of impact should be characterized by extreme tension, followed by immediate relaxation. Reducing the time during which the body exhibits tension markedly increases both the speed and the impact strength of the movement. When performed correctly, the speed and power of *fajing* can be likened to the crack of a whip, exhibiting both flexibility and "softness." Like a travelling bullet, the force should be spiralling and piercing at the same time. While Chen Taijiquan utilizes rapid shaking movement of the waist and hips during *fajing*, some practitioners over-emphasize this aspect. Shaking the body without having a fixed point of impact is of little value in practical terms. Excessive shaking may appear impressive to the untrained eye, but in terms of combat, it poses little threat to an opponent.

Chen Taijiquan *fajing* should be elastic in quality, forceful without being stiff. Its essential character is *"like a golden lion tossing its mane."* Other writers liken Taijiquan *fajing* to *"a dog shaking water from its back,"* while a Chen family saying likens it to *"shaking cinders from the back of the hand."* To be able to utilize this elastic force, the practitioner needs to develop the ability to closely co-ordinate the movement of the *yao* (waist) and *dang* (crotch). When emitting energy, the waist is turned, while simultaneously the *dang* is closed (*zhuan yao kou dang*). This ensures that as the waist spirals, the power in the *dang* is contained and not allowed to disperse. In addition to increasing the elasticity of a movement, this coordination also significantly increases its speed. The spirit of Chen Taijiquan *fajing* is reflected in the saying:

Body like a bow, hand like the arrow.
Gathering strength is like drawing the bow.
Fajing is like releasing the arrow.

When the internal energy moves from the feet to the hands, energy is issued. The more a person trains, the stronger the force will be. Those practitioners who work hard on issuing power can develop muscle extension power throughout the body. The use of explosive single movements trains one to be simultaneously loose, dynamic and extended. In summary, therefore, when preparing to *fajing*, it is necessary that the whole body ready itself. Strength is contained in both the upper and lower body, while at the same time every muscle is relaxed, loosened and sunk down. Concentration on softness is necessary in order to achieve the embodiment of the relaxed concentration of speed and maximum power, returning to relaxation immediately after power is released.

As a means to develop the ability to emit energy in the most efficient manner, *fajing* requires the practitioner to objectively evaluate a number of factors: firstly, whether or not the *jing* is initiated from the feet; secondly, whether the *yao* and *dang* spiral force is present; and thirdly, whether there is sufficient force at the point of impact. By studying the principles behind the use of *fajing*, one can increase the power and effectiveness of *fajing* movements without being sidetracked.

Consciousness lies at the heart of all Taijiquan movement. To develop a high degree of *fajing* ability there must be a close synchronization of mind intent (*yi nien*) and internal qi (*nei qi*). Following the Taijiquan classics: *"using the yi to lead the qi and using the qi to lead the body."* Immediately as the *yi* is activated, the whole body moves together. Power comes not from forced effort but is a natural manifestation of the correct alignment of the waist, hips, shoulders and back, and the efficient transference of weight.

Qinna (Seizing and Grasping)

Qinna includes grasping, seizing and locking techniques, constituting an integral component of most traditional Chinese martial arts. *Qin* is seizing or capturing the opponent to control him. If *qin* alone is used, control may be less than complete, leaving the opportunity for him to escape. *Na* is grasping the opponent to exert control over his joints. Spiralling force is used to close the joints or bend them backwards, to the point where escape or resistance is impossible. In practice, *qinna* techniques often combine several principles at once. Misplacing the bone and separating the muscle can be performed simultaneously with sealing the breath for complete control of the opponent. Many *qinna* techniques are contained within the solo forms and further developed through push hands practice. For example, *qin* is used in the movement Parting the Wild Horse's Mane, while *na* is used in Six Sealing and Four Closing.

Qinna methods from external martial arts such as *Shaolin Quan* are usually developed from a foundation of hand and arm strengthening, toughening and grip training. The effective application of the methods is often correlated to the physical strength of the practitioner. In contrast, Taijiquan's *qinna* applications are based not on physical strength but on soft internal strength, utilizing

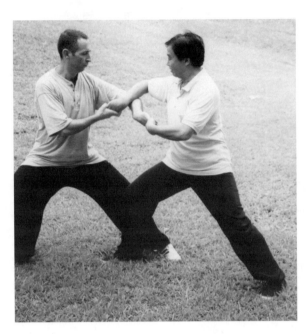

FIGURE 4.9
Zhu Tiancai
demonstrating 'qinna'
technique to
David Gaffney

mind intention and qi. By means of *"listening jing,"* the practitioner develops attunement to an opponent's reactions, responding
accordingly. When applying a *qinna* technique, movements should
be light and nimble, so that the opponent will not discern the
action and retreat from it. Grasping does not use the hands alone,
as that can be easily neutralized.

The pivot of *qinna* is in the waist and legs. When executing a
technique relax the shoulders, keep the elbows down, store the
chest, strengthen the back and concentrate the qi. Keep one's center of gravity steady, and stay close to the opponent in order to
maintain a stable stance. *Qinna* involves grasping the moving joints,
such as the wrist, elbow, shoulder, etc., so that an opponent cannot easily escape. In Chen Taijiquan there are numerous ways to
make the opponent's qi rise up, one of which is *qinna*. When qi
rises, the root (balance) is compromised, and the person can be
easily taken down. It also renders the chest area vulnerable to
strikes.

When developing *qinna* skills, it is not always necessary to take joint-locks and takedowns to the point of completion. The goal should be to become familiar with the principles and techniques. Practicing co-operatively with a partner allows both to realize the skill while protecting the body's joints from unnecessary injury.

Push Hands

To bridge the gap between form and free fighting, Chen Wangting devised the unique Taijiquan push hands exercises. Perhaps the most important reason for practicing push hands is to develop sensitivity to the movement of a partner or opponent, and to be able to respond appropriately to any incoming force. Many Taiji students are too anxious to start doing push hands, often beginning before they have learned to do the form and solo exercises proficiently. It is important to realize that form training will provide a solid foundation upon which to subsequently build good push hands skills. Most of the techniques used in push hands can be found in the form. Push hands is covered in detail in Chapter Five.

Equipment Training

Past generations of masters placed great importance upon special power training methods *(xing gong)*, pole-shaking *(dou gunzi)*, Taiji ruler *(xing gong bang)*, Taiji ball and the use of sandbags. *Zhan zhuang*, forms practice, silk-reeling exercises, push hands, etc., all lead to an increase in internal strength. At a more advanced stage, the use of supplementary exercises with a variety of training aids can further develop this energy. Skills such as neutralizing, yielding, *qinna* and *fajing* are more efficient when supported by strength. Furthermore, certain movements within the Taiji form are difficult to practice safely with a partner. Supplementary exercise training allows these movements to be developed to their full potential.

Pole-Shaking

Cut from the baila tree, the long pole is usually approximately four yards long and about an inch and a half in diameter. This type of wood is flexible and springy, allowing the practitioner to transmit force through it. Hardwood or metal poles are unsuitable, as they lack this elasticity. Shaking the long pole is an effective way to enhance and develop the dantian's ability to issue power and transmit it to the hands and feet. Various actions can be practiced, such as lifting, covering, thrusting and shaking.

There are several different ways of training with the long pole. The most common method is as follows: Assuming a bow stance, the practitioner holds the pole facing forward obliquely. That is, if the left leg is forward, the pole points towards the right front corner. The left hand grips the end of the pole closest to the body, while the right extends towards the center. To perform the drill, the weight is shifted onto the back leg while the pole circles back and then up. At this point, the weight is forcefully shifted and sunk

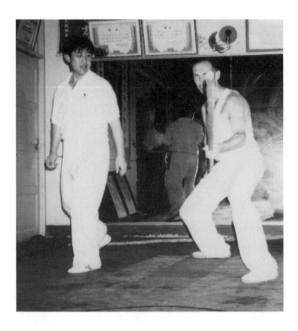

FIGURE 4.10
David Gaffney training with the long pole under the supervision of Chen Zhenglei

into the front leg and the front hand pushes out and down.

Throughout the movement, the hand gripping the end of the pole remains close to the body. When performing the pole-shaking exercise, it is important that the practitioner emits power through the tip of the pole. In practical terms this means that the end of the pole should vibrate with each energy release. In practice, the *fajing* can be performed during either the opening or closing phase of the movement. Training with the long pole can greatly increase the power of the waist and arms, as well as the body's elastic shaking power. Along with performing at least thirty sets of boxing, seventeenth-generation master Chen Fa-ke was reputed to do three hundred repetitions of the pole-shaking exercise daily.

Taiji Ball

The Taiji ball is a metal ball roughly equal in size to a basketball. Chen Taijiquan requires the internal qi to propel the external form. By turning and rolling the Taiji ball, the practitioner seeks to initiate movement from the dantian so that the turning of the sphere simply reflects the movement of an invisible ball within the abdomen. This feeling is described in the Chen family's "Song of the Taiji Ball":

> Training in the eighteen methods with the Taiji sphere,
> the method never strays from circles of silk twining.
> Changing in infinite permutations of Yin and Yang energy,
> a perfectly round shape is formed internally.

During push hands practice or martial applications, the body's "internal sphere" (dantian) rotates according to the external force applied. Practice with the Taiji ball allows the practitioner to turn the dantian naturally, and upon encountering an outside force, to move the entire body in response.

A common exercise uses one hand to hold the ball and roll it up and down against the wall. This allows one to develop the upward silk-reeling strength, as well as increase the force in the lower body, waist, shoulders and wrists. Over time, the flexibility of the fingers and palm increases, improving ability in *qinna* as well as pushing techniques.

Taiji *Bang* (Stick)

Rolling dough to make *jiaozi* (Beijing dumplings) for her family, the wife of Chen Fa-ke inadvertently provided the inspiration for her husband to devise the Taiji *bang*. San Francisco-based Chen Taijiquan teacher Zhang Xuexin, a student of Chen Zhaokui and Feng Zhiqiang, tells how Chen Fa-ke was suddenly struck by the idea that twisting the short rolling pin she was using would be an excellent way to train the *qinna* skills of Taijiquan.

Chen Fa-ke's youngest son, Chen Zhaokui, further developed the Taiji *bang* by making the ends of the stick slightly thinner than the middle and rounding them off. This allowed the person train-

FIGURE 4.11
Davidine Sim and Zhang Xuexin 'Twisting the Taiji Bang'

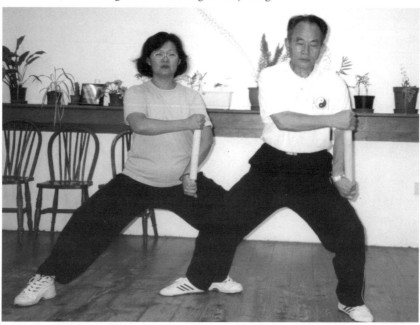

ing with the Taiji *bang* to be able to turn the wrists more flexibly, simulating grasping and neutralizing movements. Rounding off the ends allows them to fit comfortably into the *Laogong* points in the center of the palms. Chen Zhaokui was renowned for his *qinna* skills and, of all the supplementary equipment, favored "Wringing the Stick" *(Ning Bang Zi)*.

Using a short stick roughly equal to the forearm in length and thickness, the Taiji practitioner can significantly improve the strength of their grip, wrists, elbows and shoulders. The method involves manipulating the stick through the use of whole-body circular movement to practice *qinna* and counter-*qinna* actions. Numerous movements within the Chen Taiji form are *qinna* techniques. Thus practicing the Taiji *bang* helps not only to develop general *qinna* skills, but also to understand the correct hand positioning in the form.

As one grips the stick tightly, various hand positions are practiced. For example, both hands gripping with palms facing downwards is considered to be yang-yang *bang,* palms upward represents yin-yin *bang,* etc. When using the Taiji *bang,* emphasis should be upon developing the flexibility and twisting strength of the wrists and elbows, as well as the ability to fold the chest and waist. Consistent practice increases the stability and rooting strength of the legs and enhances the ability to freely open and close the shoulders and *kua.*

Traditionally, Taiji exponents are asked to *"use yi not li,"* that is, to use mind intent rather than physical strength. Often interpreted as meaning that no physical force should be used, a more accurate interpretation would be to use mind rather than stiff untrained force that can be readily manipulated by an opponent. For beginners, the most important thing is to rid oneself of stiffness. At this stage relaxation and loosening of the body are emphasized rather than strength training. Once the ability to use internal force has been developed, then strength training can be practiced with no negative effect on relaxation. Above all practice must be patient, diligent and persistent if an advanced level of ability is to be attained. To quote an old Chinese proverb: "One day's chill does not result in three feet of ice" (*bing dong san che, fei yi zhe zi han*).

CHAPTER FIVE

Push Hands (*Tui Shou*)

Created by Chen Wangting, push hands is a composite practice method by which the Taiji form is put to use. It acts as a bridge linking form training to applications, and is a way of learning the combative and defensive skills of the art. Originally known as "hitting hands" (*da shou*) or "crossing hands" (*ke shou*), it is a method formulated by the combination of Taiji principles and the martial methods of grasping, wrestling and throwing. Push hands has further developed and improved to become a unique style in its own right.

The core of the method is the spirals of *chan ssu jing* combined with twining, coiling, sticking and following movements, based on the concept of the Taiji polarity. As mentioned before, Taijiquan is based on the ancient theory of the two opposing and yet complementing forces of yin and yang. It requires stillness as well as movement; softness as well as hardness; lightness and steadiness; insubstantial and substantial; slowness and speed. In this way yin never departs from yang nor yang from yin. Yang force results from yin and vice versa.

The aim of Taijiquan practice is to reach a stage whereby a balance of the two forces is achieved, where both forces appear simultaneously. The skill is then further developed to a stage when yin and yang can no longer be discerned. In Taiji form and push hands practice, therefore, movements should be a balance of both yin and yang. In order to be recognized as Taijiquan there must exist the ability to be soft as well as hard; the presence of lightness as well

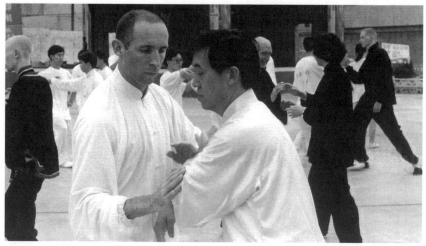

FIGURE 5.1 David Gaffney pushing hands with Chen Zhenglei in Zhengzhou, China.

as solidity; a clear differentiation of full and empty; a combination of stillness and motion; and the capability to react to attack with speed and to adhere with ease.

Push hands is the mutual exploration of the internal energies and is dependent primarily on the sense of touch. The method involves two people making contact at the arms, adhering to each other, using the Taiji spiral movements. It is based on the principles of *"adhering and following, neither let go nor resist."* This concept means connecting and joining *(zhan lien)* on a vertical plane, and sticking and following *(nien sui)* on a horizontal plane. Not letting go *(pu tiu)* means not losing contact with the opponent's arm, and not resisting *(pu ding)* means not opposing him. This enables a person to develop sensitivity of the whole body, from the skin to the internal core, in order to discern the subtlest change in the opponent and to react instantly to it.

Push hands has the Taiji form as its foundation, with the usege of relaxed skill. But contained within it are methods that need to be understood. There are certain rules that must be observed. Pushing hands, like practicing the form, utilizes the eight energies *(jing)* of the body. These are *peng* (warding), *lu* (diverting), *ji* (squeezing), *an* (pressing down), considered as the primary energies; and *cai* (plucking), *lie* (splitting), *zhou* (elbowing), *kao* (bumping), seen as subsidiary energies. Emphasis is also put on the five directions: *jin* (advance), *tui* (retreat), *zuo-gu* (guard left), *you-pan* (anticipate right) and *zhong-ding* (central equilibrium).

The five directions are usually regarded as footwork, but they are more than that. They are also the mind intent on, or the awareness of, one's position and that of the opponent's in relation to the five directions. The emphasis in push hands is not pushing an opponent over, but seeking out the opponent's and one's own center of equilibrium and the perimeter of stability. This knowledge enables both parties to learn to stay within their boundary of stability and balance, and also to learn how they can extend the range of effective perimeter. This can only be achieved through mutual co-operation during practice.

When pushing hands, it is important to "relax" *(song)* and to "invest in loss." It is worth keeping in mind that only one component of push hands is pushing. Yielding is the other. It is described as *zhou*, moving away. When pushed on the left side, for example, one should empty that side by yielding or moving away. It may not be easy to follow this ultimately rewarding path, as the tendency is to defend by resisting. The key is to adhere to the other person and follow the force of the push with sensitivity, all the time keeping one's root. This way it will be possible to learn to gauge oncoming force, and to discover the infinite number of methods by which to yield to the varieties of pushes. In other words, to discover all the boundaries of one's limits and to create ways of protecting them.

There should be a constant interchange of yin (soft and yielding) and yang (firm and advancing). The aim is not just to get the better of your push hands partner, but also to achieve a balance of yin and yang energies. If a person continues to yield when being pushed and does not know the boundary of the yield, balance will be lost. Yielding leads to neutralizing *(hua)*. Neutralizing should be a part of every technique, involving the absorption of another's energy to become like a compressed spring. This reduces one's own center and makes it undetectable, and the borrowed energy can then be issued back. The technique can take two forms—one is to attune with the opponent's movement and entice him further in order to take advantage of his position; the other is to feign weakness, causing him to commit himself rashly. Chen Xin's *Boxing Treatise* said, "Entice the opponent with an 'empty basket'; then just make one turn." The "Song of Pushing Hands" stated, "Lure the opponent into emptiness; harmonize with him, then emit [force]."

In practice, emitting force *(fajing)* is not the use of stiff, forceful energy. For example, in push hands practice, attacking movements could be warding off *(peng)* or squeezing *(ji)*. Likewise, "soft" should not be the softness that is weak and limp, but one that has the significance of conserving, protecting or guarding *(shou)*. Examples could be the defensive movements of diverting *(lu)* or pressing down *(an)*. In both attack and defense, therefore, the "hard" and "soft" are dependent on mind intent and inner consciousness.

Ba Fa—The Eight Kinetic Movements of Taijiquan

Ba means "eight." *Fa* means "methods." *Ba fa* involves the eight trained energies of the body *(jing)*, from which all skills and techniques are generated. It is also the eight hand-skill methods of Taijiquan, and the main idea in push hands. It is the most fundamental study in Chen style.

The four frontal methods *(si zheng)* are *peng* (warding), *lu* (diverting), *ji* (squeezing) and *an* (pressing down), which represent the four main directions and are derived from the vertical circle. *Zheng* means "fixed or unchangeable" and is therefore not influenced by others.

The four diagonal methods *(si yu)* are *cai* (plucking), *lie* (splitting), *zhou* (elbowing) and *kao* (bumping), which represent the four secondary directions and are derived from the horizontal circle. *Yu* means "diagonal or sideways" and is changeable. These supplement and assist the four frontal methods.

Peng

Taijiquan has been called *Peng Jin Quan* or "Peng Energy Boxing" as described in the famous Chen book by Gu Liuxin and Shen Jiazheng.

Peng carries two meanings. The first is a sense of buoyancy throughout the body, giving it a feeling of vitality and resilience (*nei qi*). It is contained in every movement at all times and is an inflated, outward-expanding energy. The second is an action, a technique that uses a vertical circular movement that spirals upwards and outwards, intercepting and warding off an advancing force.

Peng energy is created by the elastic force of muscles, combined with the elongation of the joints and tendons. It can be compared with the buoyancy of water. On it a tiny leaf can drift, but it can also carry a ten-thousand-ton ship. *Peng* energy prevents an opponent from reaching one's body. The *peng* strength used never exceeds the strength an opponent is using in attack. It is sufficient only to hold off an attack, but not to resist or stop the attack. The main purpose is to prevent the opponent from reaching one's body and then to change the direction of the attack by utilizing one of the other hand methods. *Peng* energy, therefore, acts as the foundation for the change of energies in push hands.

As it is an organic (living) force, it can only be truly felt and realized in push hands. It is difficult for those who have never pushed hands to fully understand this concept. Proper understanding of the concept and acquisition of the authentic skill cannot be achieved by attempts at logic or theoretical guessing. Only through diligent and consistent as well as intelligent practice can one reach a level of proficiency.

Example of *peng:* Transition from Single Whip (*Dan Bian*) to Buddha's Warrior Attendant Pounds Mortar (Jin Gang *Dao Dui*).

Lu

Lu is a diverting action. It involves an oblique drawing movement, which can go upwards or downwards in a horizontal circular plane. The aim of the *lu* energy is to *"direct an opponent's energy towards emptiness."* It is important to note that *lu* is not a pulling energy. It follows the opponent's energy in order to move him with a slight change of direction, thus unloading his force from one's own body. This method is frequently used to neutralize *peng.*

Example of *lu:* Transition from Lazily Tying Coat (*Lan Zha Yee*) to Six Sealing and Four Closing (*Liu Feng Si Bi*).

Ji

Ji is utilized when an opponent's energy is going backwards. It follows the withdrawing energy, using a horizontal spiral movement to crowd or squeeze into the opponent's center. *Ji* is used to spoil *lu* energy. It can force a guarding opponent to commit and is used in both defense and attack. The method can be executed with double hands, single hand, arms, shoulders and the body, depending on the distance of the opponent. Good balance is necessary for effective use of the method.

Example of *ji:* Lazily Tying Coat (*Lan Zha Yee*) .

An

An is an upward then downward energy, done in a vertical circular pattern. *An* is the most frequently used method in Taijiquan. It creates a feeling of pressure, effectively sealing and closing an opponent's energy, and is carried out by emptying the chest and pressing downward. It is used in attack but is also a good defensive move. It is often used to destroy *ji* energy.

Example of *an:* Beginning Posture (*Qi Shi*).

Peng-lu-ji-an can be said to be all variations of the *peng* energy, which is present in all postures and movements. *Peng* is expressed in *lu, ji* and *an* in that *lu* is considered a backward *peng, ji* is a forward *peng*, and *an* is a downward *peng*. The importance of understanding these energies is expressed in the saying: "You must differentiate and pay attention to *peng-lu-ji-an*; coordination of the upper and lower body prevents an opponent from entering" *(Peng lu ji an xu ren zhen; shang xia xiang shui ren nan jin)*.

Cai

Cai indicates an energy that changes the direction of an opponent's incoming force. *Cai* applies a lever action by calculating an incoming force and integrating it with one's own energy whilst redirecting, so that the balance scales of equilibrium are tipped in one's favor. The main action is done with the fingers to control an opponent's lower arm, using the twist of the waist to generate power. The energy is short and swift, using small circular movement. It is important to keep the shoulders and elbows down and have *jing* concentrated in them. The technique can be used within the processes of *lu* and *an*.

Example of *cai:* Forward and Backward Trick *(Qian Zhao, Hou Zhao)*.

Lie

Lie is a rending action executed from the waist, with the rotation of the upper arm/shoulder area working in harmony with the centerline. Two opposing forces are applied to cause imbalance. The waist has to be flexible, utilizing the silk-reeling spiral in execution. This is a rapid emptying (dodging) movement made in the process of being seized, causing an opponent to lose balance, and then the moment is used to launch an offensive. *Lie* is a quick-release "surprise" that startles an opponent both physically and mentally. This move typifies *"four ounces overcomes a thousand pounds."*

Example of *lie:* Drape Fist Over Body *(Pie Shen Quan)*.

Zhou

Zhou is using the elbows to attack. It can be done in many different planes—horizontal, vertical, rising, swinging. It is a short strike within the reach of the elbow. *Zhou* is considered to be the second line of defense. As the saying goes: *"When far use the hands, when near use the elbows."* The elbow is a very effective weapon, usually directed at the upper torso, which can cause serious injury. In study push hands, the tip of the elbow should not be used.

Example of *zhou:* Green Dragon Out of the Water (*Qing Lung Chu Shui*).

Kao

The use of *kao* is one of the specialities of Taijiquan and is not easy to master. It involves close-range control of energy. *Kao* basically means to lean or to bump. *Kao* motions are often referred to as shoulder strikes, but it can also be elbow *kao*, knee *kao*, hip *kao*, etc., using the shoulders, chest, hips, or back. *Kao* can be executed with straightforward shifting or with added rotation. The skill of the technique lies with the shoulders and back and offers the element of *beng* (bursting) force. Taking the above saying a step further: *"When far use the hands, when near use the elbows. When close to the body use kao and there will be no escape."* *Kao* is the core energy expressed in *cai-lie-zhou-kao*, just as *peng* is the core energy for the first four. Whenever and wherever you make contact, there is *kao*.

Example of *kao:* Diagonal Step (*Xie Xing*).

The four frontal methods use relatively longer forces, while the four diagonal methods are shorter forces (inch force) and are more explosive. The *ba fa* are training methods for understanding the energies of the body. The first step is to study the movements correctly, where the energies are obvious *(ming-jing)*. In advanced study one should focus on the internal details, as movements are always led by the mind *(an-jing)*.

Body movement skills are closely linked with footwork skills, and the two need to be combined.

Wu Bu—The Five Footwork Skills of Taijiquan

Wu means "five" and *bu* means "steps." *Wu bu* is considered the foundation of *ba fa*, because hand skills can only work efficiently if the body moves into the right position. The five footwork skills are as follows:

Jin (**Advance**)—to go forward or to step into. This is to close into an opponent directly.

Tui (**Retreat**)—to move backward or to step back. This is to withdraw one's body directly in order to create a distance between oneself and the opponent.

Zuo-Gu (**Guard Left**)—to advance sideways. As opposed to *jin* that goes forward directly, *zuo-gu* closes up to an opponent indirectly. In this context, *zuo* (left) means "sideways." *Gu* means "to guard against, to be careful." It is defensiveness within attack.

You-Pan (**Anticipate Right**)—to retreat sideways. Here *you* means "sideways" and *pan* means "anticipating, looking out for." It is defensiveness within retreat.

Zuo-gu and *you-pan* also train the responsive motions of the eyes to observe the opponent's every move.

Zhong-Ding (**Central Equilibrium**)—to maintain balance and stability. The main idea is to create a point of energy or strength which is straight and balanced, so that the body is ready to do anything. *Zhong-ding*, from the top of the head through the body to a point in between the feet, is like a single post that must not be allowed to move off-center. This alignment needs to be sought internally as well as externally. It is invisible and used inside, not outside.

The correct execution of Chen form and push hands involves

the development of *zhong-ding*, which maintains stability throughout all movements and postures. Every posture and stance has its inherent center, whether stationary or leaning forward or backward. To remain constantly rooted and stable, the center of gravity should be as low as possible.

Push Hands Requirements

Correct Body Posture

The body is kept upright and not leaning. Relax the neck to gently support the head. The chest is "contained" (slightly concave) and the back is naturally straight. Qi sinks down to the dantian. The tailbone is centered so that the *Baihui* point on the crown of the head lines up with the *Huiyin* point in between the legs. This straight line should be maintained throughout. Each section of the vertebrae should be relaxed and yet connected. The waist is settled but flexible, not collapsed or unsteady. The waist plays a crucial part in keeping the body's central equilibrium, both in posture and in motion, and serves to support all "eight directions." Counterbalance is provided by the *Mingmen*. For example, when arms and legs move forward, the *Mingmen* draws back, regulating balance and maintaining central equilibrium. *Mingmen* is also the initiation point of power release in the waist. Its appropriate usage is extremely important in determining the effectiveness of pushing hands. The change from substantial (weight-bearing) to insubstantial (non-weight-bearing) stances also relies on the use of the waist and *Mingmen*. Here they act as the axis to turn the loin area. For example, as the left loin contracts and draws in, the left side becomes substantial and the right side becomes insubstantial.

Taiji push hands requires the correct use of the body, as well as the push hands principles of *"connect, join, stick and follow"*; *"neither let go nor resist."* When a partner uses *an* (press down), you *peng* (ward off). When he uses *ji* (squeeze in), you *lu* (divert away). With continuous and consistent practice, a solid foundation of Taijiquan will be established. In both Taiji form and push hands the correct body posture is of utmost importance, as a good body alignment allows one to control others and yet prevent others from entering one's perimeter. The "Song of Pushing Hands" says, *"Be conscientious about* peng, lu, ji, an. *Following each other above and below, difficult for people to enter."* The famous fourteenth-generation Chen ancestor Chen Changxing was famous for his upright posture, earning the nickname "Ancestral Tablet."

Before beginning the practice of push hands, one must understand correct movement principles. Most important is whole-body movement. Once the dantian moves, the whole body moves. When the coordination of the whole body is understood, then one will not use only the upper body to push hands, or just use the hands and arms to push.

Hand Technique

The hands function as the antennae to pick up energy and should be free of tension. Taiji push hands requires that one *"know oneself and know the opponent."* The first skill of push hands, therefore, is to train sensitivity. On each hand there are nine "antennae" or energy points: the five fingers, the two sides of the palm (*yu ji*), the center of the palm and the back of the hand. Counting both hands, therefore, there are eighteen points by which to make contact. The role of the hands is most obvious in the execution of a movement. They guide the movements of the arms. The shoulder joints must always be kept relaxed and flexible. Elbow joints are very slightly drawn in. They should be held with *yi* (mind intent) and not *li* (strength) at all times. This requirement is very important, in both neutralizing and advancing, in order not to divulge to the opponent one's intended move.

For beginners, the silk-reeling circles are bigger and more expansive. As much as possible one should maintain a smooth flow so that the circular movements are full and not deflated or broken at any point. Use mind intent *(yi)* together with energy *(jing)* and not strength *(li)*. Do not push back or resist incoming energy. Movements should be slow and deliberate, as it is easy to lose sight of body requirements and principles in fast, uncontrolled movements. As one's skill increases, one gradually reduces the circle. Tempo can then be flexible and adaptable, according to the speed of incoming energies.

In practice, movements should be light and relaxed at the beginning. Experienced practitioners can progress to the heavy, sunken-type movements. The palms and wrists are the contact points for controlling the arms of the opponent, limiting the movements of his lower wrist section, the middle elbow section and the upper shoulder section to make them ineffective. There is also the additional possibility of *qinna* (seizing and locking).

Footwork

In movements, the footwork must be light and agile. This is possible through the understanding of proper weight distribution and weight change. It is the ability to differentiate the substantial (weight-bearing) and insubstantial (non-weight-bearing) in each posture. Chen Xin says in his Taijiquan treatises: "If you are single-weighted, you can be responsive. If you are double-weighted, you are stagnant." In the practice of push hands, these two sentences are very important. "Double-weighted" does not mean having equal weight on both legs. If it were that simple, as Chen Xiaowang says, then one needs only to shift more weight to one side to correct it. "Double-weighted" means that the Taiji yin-yang is not correct and there is stagnation of qi in a static posture. In push hands, one's movement is stifled by an opponent and there is no scope for change. A practitioner can only have a superficial understanding of Taijiquan if he/she does not understand this concept.

In order for the footwork to be agile, the *kua* must be flexible and relaxed. This is made possible by the close coordination of the waist and *kua*. Remember that the body leads all movements. Weight changes must be smooth and natural, with the correct principle of folding the waist and relaxing the *kua*. The substantial leg should be spiralled into the ground, with mind intent a fraction deeper into the ground. This creates a firm, unshakeable stance and posture that cannot be upset in any way. In advance the *kua* should relax first, then in an arc movement one advances slightly upward and forward, all the time co-ordinating with the spiral movement in the advancing arm.

Footwork is linked to hand movement, so that there is never disconnection between the lower and upper body. The "three connections" (*san he*) denote the connections of the palms with the feet, the elbows with the knees and the shoulders with the *kua*.

With a firm and solid stance, the substantial foot must be fully on the ground, neither tilting one way nor the other. The toes grip the ground, and it is this that makes *fajing* (emitting energy) more effective. The ground can serve as a "kickboard" when the heel pushes against it. Thus *"energy is generated in the feet, controlled by the waist, transmitted through the back, and manifested in the hands."* In properly executed weight shifts the force can go straight through to the opponent's feet and uproot him.

In push hands, an advance invariably involves stepping in or entering into the opponent's space. Stepping in involves the techniques of "hook" (*tau*) and "plant" (*qa*). They can also be explained as encompassing or penetrating steps, respectively. To *tau* is to use the front foot to closely press onto the outside of the opponent's front foot, thereby restricting and controlling his movement—encompassing an opponent by stepping around his stance. To *qa* is to plant one's front foot in the space between the opponent's legs, thereby intimidating him—penetrating the opponent's stance at the point of weight distribution. Elbow and shoulder strikes use *qa* or penetrating steps. The encompassing *tau* and penetrating *qa* are therefore the two most commonly used methods to gain advantage position in push hands. The knees are used similarly when inward turn and outward tilt movements are executed with elastic energy to uproot and fell an opponent (can also be used for neutralizing an opponent's attempt at uprooting you). Chen style Taiji push hands continues to retain the goal of felling opponents. Chen Xin states, *"Boxing is simply for felling; to not understand this is exertion in vain."*

Eye Technique

The eyes are known as the window of the soul. In Chinese martial arts, the eyes play a key role. It is said that the brain commands and the eyes convey.

The expression of the eyes is in accordance with the movement. Each movement is led by *yi* (mind). The eyes follow *yi*, and these bring about reactions in the body, and the four limbs. Therefore, the direction of eye gaze should not be independent from a movement. In other words, the eyes and the mind intent are consistent. They are alert, focused and ever-watchful—guarding every direction and anticipating each move. If the eyes and the movements are not co-ordinated, then it can be said that there is no connection between the internal and external. Taking this a step further, in combat the eyes are used in relation to an opponent's movements.

The sense of sight is vital when assessing an opportunity or opening for advance or attack. This opportunity usually arises when the opponent loses control of his center of mass. The eyes provide the speed in seeing opportunities, and they supplement the sense of touch. Having seen the opening, it is also necessary to ascertain where the weakness is, and the direction from which to attack. If the position and direction are not assessed and settled quickly, you will allow the opponent to regain control. Therefore, while it is important to rely on the sense of touch in push hands for *ting jing* (listening to energy), the use of the eyes is equally valuable.

The eyes are also used for intimidation. A steady gaze full of intent can often make an opponent less confident and more apprehensive and fearful, thus weakening his position while strengthening one's own. The method of the eyes must be natural, neither staring nor wandering, with the spirit held within. The eyes should not be opened too wide so as to let the opponent read one's intention. Nor, obviously, should the eyes be closed.

Many practitioners rely solely on the sense of touch to develop their skills. Very often they turn their heads aside while pushing hands, or close their eyes. This is a mistake. There should be a combination and coordination of sight, hearing and touch, and one is not exclusive of the others.

Adhere and Follow *(Zhan Lian Nian Sui)*

Zhan *is an energy that finds and connects with a partner's energy.*
Lian *is an energy that links and joins with a partner's energy.*
Nian *adheres to and merges with a partner's energy.*
Sui *follows and pursues a partner's energy.*

One does not just adhere and follow with the hands, but also with the body and footwork. The whole body must work as a tight unit, with no separation or disconnection of any part. Only then can one adhere and draw the opponent in order to control him. Do not pre-plan a course of action but simply follow the opponent's movements closely—*"forget self to follow others" (she ji cong ren)*. Move forward as he retreats; withdraw as he advances; connect and merge with his actions; and it will be possible to discern his intention and use it to one's advantage. This is *"dong jing"* or understanding energy. Focus on the opponent's motion to gauge the direction of his incoming energy and the precise position of his center of balance. Your response and action must be totally dependent on his. *Dong jing* is the ability to clearly distinguish between the positive and negative and to react accordingly in order to take full advantage of the changes. "Know your opponent as you know yourself, a hundred battles bring a hundred victories," wrote Sun Zi in *The Art of War (Bing Fa)*. Generally, use *zhan* and *nian* energies to find the opportunity to put an opponent in an unfavorable position. *Lian* and *sui* are skills for getting out of a predicament presented by an opponent.

A quiet and still mind is necessary for *ting jing* or the ability to listen to an opponent's energy. Listening *jing* is essential to understanding changes in the opponent's movement. With this will come the knowledge of when and how to react. It is part of relaxing the body. In push hands agility, and flexibility are essential, and power comes from internal relaxation. When the mind is tense, sensitivity to oneself as well as external forces is limited.

Neutralizing Skill

In push hands practice, the tendency of most people is to keep a partner at bay. This is especially so for the practitioners with some physical strength. The main emphasis will be to hold off a partner using strength that is sustained beyond its usefulness, thereby committing the cardinal fault of resisting *(ding jing)*. When this happens, an important aspect of push hands, neutralizing *(hua jing)*, is overlooked. The skill of push hands lies in detecting and neutralizing force, not resisting force. Neutralizing skill requires soft *jing* (soft energy), the opposite of *fajing* (emitting force). *Fajing* is issuing force at the right moment, and *hua jing* is interpreting and neutralizing force at the right moment. In both instances, timing is crucial.

The first requirement is to welcome a partner's force in, and not to make the first move. True neutralizing occurs when one goes with the direction of the opponent's incoming force, then changes its direction by responding when the opportunity presents itself. The opportunity may arise when the opponent has over-extended and is at the point of losing balance, just before he retreats. Use the momentum to unbalance him. Or take advantage when the opponent's *jing* is about to surface, yet has not completely emerged. At the instant when the force is about to arrive, follow it and neutralize. The key is to use the other's momentum to react. Too early or too fast, and there is nothing to neutralize. Too late or too slow, and the opportunity has passed.

Neutralization should be a part of every technique. For example, neutralize before executing a *qinna* (grasp and lock). At a higher level of skill, one can advance while neutralizing. For example, the upper body retreats and neutralizes while the lower body moves in to attack; or one can neutralize linearly while attacking laterally. This is known as advancing by retreating. A beginner is only able to use neutralizing as a mean of escape. To develop the true skill of neutralization requires constant practice and experimentation. One must not focus one's mind only on winning, using unnecessary force to hold off a partner, or be in a hurry to emit force to topple a partner. One must "invest in loss" and put aside misplaced pride, arrogance and the concern for "losing face." The practitioner may be uprooted and unbalanced many times before being able to instinctively absorb and redirect an incoming force to any part of one's body. Neutralizing is not done with the hands and shoulders, but with the waist and legs. Begin with bigger circles to neutralize. The higher one's skill, the smaller the circle will be.

Awareness of Opportunity

Awareness of opportunity is developed over time, through diligent practice to increase and refine sensitivity and reactions.

Wu Kongcho's discourse on Wu Style (1930) contains observations of push hands which are equally applicable to all styles. He notes the three levels of skill in push hands are Non-Awareness; Awareness After the Fact; and Awareness Before the Fact.

At the moment when yin and yang have yet to surface, when inactivity and activity are not yet apparent, and substantial and insubstantial are indistinct, there is a brief instant of prescience. This is opportunity. Only the experienced are alert to it and able to manipulate the situation to their advantage, creating something from nothing. The inexperienced do not have this ability. The consummate maintains calmness and grace as he handles the incoming opposing force. The inexperienced finds no means to advance or retreat. This the fundamental difference between awareness and non-awareness of opportunity.

Types of Push Hands

Push hands can be divided into the study-type push hands and the competitive-type push hands. While sharing the same format, the determining concept is entirely different. The emphasis of the study type is to research how Taiji theory and principle can be applied in actuality and to raise one's level of understanding and skill. Victory or defeat is outside its context. The main focus is on sharpening the senses and developing the ability to feel internal energy. Competitive push hands is guided by a mind that is set on winning. There can never be too much deception in war, but the aim is on winning with skill and intelligence. "In War let your great object be victory, not lengthy campaigns," wrote Sun Zi in *The Art of War (Bing Fa)*.

In Chen style, there are five types of Push Hands:

- *Wuan Hua*— fixed step—single- and double-handed exercises
- *Ding Bu*—fixed step—double-handed
- *Huang Bu (jin yi tui yi)*—single backward/forward step— double-handed
- *Da Lu*—moving step—low stance—double-handed
- *Luang Cai Hua*—free steps—double-handed

Beyond these is the practice of san *tui* or free pushing.

Wuan hua ("Reeling flowers") utilizes the shoulders to drive the arms in three directions, using *shun-chan, ni-chan,* inward-*chan* and outward-*chan* of the silk-reeling movements. The exercise concentrates on the opening and closing movements of the torso and the hips. Students should pay attention to the basic requirements of sinking the *kua*, turning the waist, and opening and closing the chest. It is also practiced to develop listening skills *(ting jing)*.

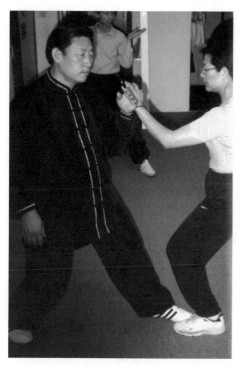

Although seemingly simple to perform, this exercise, if done correctly, teaches the proper coordination of the lower and upper body. It trains awareness of posture, relaxation, sensitivity, leg usage, motor skills and torso-related technical application.

Ding bu means "fixed step." It involves more physical contact that engages both partners' hands to cover the forearms and elbows. Turning the arms in vertical circles, the basic movements of *peng, lu, ji* and *an* are applied, particularly *Peng* and *An*. Listening skill is further developed, along with the sense of timing—knowledge of when, where and how to use some of the basic techniques. "Moving away" movements are practiced. *Ding bu* reveals the possibility of *qinna*, the seizing and locking skill that is highly developed in Chen style Taiji.

Huang bu means "changing steps." This exercise involves moving backward and forward with one step *(jin yi tui yi)*. The techniques of *cai, lie, zhou* and *kao* are introduced and practiced, as well

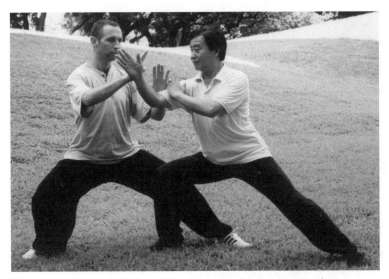

FIGURE 5.3 David Gaffney and Zhu Tiancai—Moving Step tuishou

as the first four energies. Methods of neutralizing are contained in this exercise. Although these techniques can also be found in the fixed-step push hands, *huang bu* have movements designed specifically for the practice of these techniques. *Qinna* skill is further explored and sensitivity further developed. When one is familiar

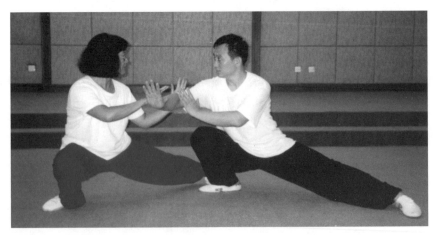

FIGURE 5.4 Davidine Sim doing Da Lu

with the movements, the stepping can be increased to three or five steps backward and forward. This stage can be used to test one's understanding of Taiji principles.

Da Lu ("big rollback") is a physically demanding technique that requires the practitioners to go down into very low postures while doing the double circular actions of *huang bu*. This training method increases the legs and torso strength, trains flexibility of footwork, and develops rooting and balance in application. The body requirements should be strictly adhered to while doing this exercise, so that qi is not dispersed in the attempt to maintain the low posture

Luang cai hua ("free-flowing steps") allows for more sponta-neous, active and flexible practice. The multiple stepping in varied directions is co-ordinated with the earlier pushing method. At this stage of training smaller steps are used. The practitioner moves freely in flexible techniques that include nimble footwork, *qinna* and neutralization, utilizing all the eight energies competently.

Beyond the five methods, martial application and combat abil-ity are further developed by the practice of *san tui* (free pushing). It bridges the gap between the form and free fighting. It allows the use of any technique learned from the Taiji form and push hands. *San tui* is akin to free sparring but is more controlled. It trains application and usage for technical familiarity and sensitivity. Usage practice also seeks to develop opponent control and neu-tralization skill (*zhouhua*). Taiji skill is incomplete if only attacking skill and emitting power are practiced but not the ability to *zhouhua* (evade and neutralize) and to lead an opponent into emptiness (*yin jin luo kong*).

Push hands, therefore, is Taijiquan's other content—mutually complementing, supplementing, enforcing and completing. Chen Zhaokui said, "Taijiquan is the foundation of push hands; and push hands is a means to test your Taiji skill." Mistakes in the form, such as lifting the shoulders and elbows, using unnecessary force, and lack of *peng* energy (a collapsed, flaccid form) will be exposed when doing push hands. Therefore, push hands is a valu-

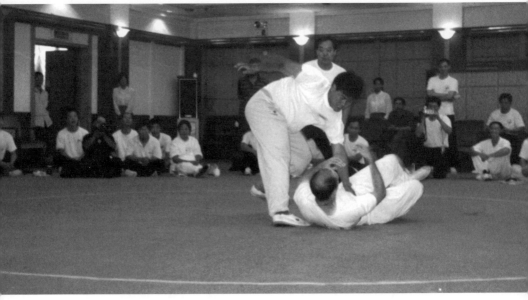

FIGURE 5.5 Competitive Push Hands

able training method whereby students can learn the reason why they have to adhere to strict principles. Push hands can be considered a kind of cultured fighting art. The form is more polished, the content more abundant. As one strives for precision, resisting coarseness, the focus is on combat with skill and intellect.

CHAPTER SIX

Weapons

Chen style Taijiquan was originally practiced, first and foremost, to build martial and military skills. While the training obviously enhanced the health of the Taiji boxers, this was not the primary reason for practicing the art. In the days of Chen Wangting, there were no guns. Traditional weapons were still being carried onto the battlefield and used in actual combat. Today, the weapon forms of the various Chinese martial arts are viewed by many only in in the context of demonstrating or exercising in the park. Considering the Chen weapon forms in this manner can only lead to a superficial understanding of their essence. Preserved within each of the Chen weapon routines is the original martial intent. In addition to showing relaxed flowing movements, the forms contain many dynamic actions, rapid changes in tempo, and ferocious chopping, slicing or thrusting movements.

Weapons training complements the barehanded practice of the Chen Taijiquan practitioner by amplifying certain requirements. For example, the mind and intention must be extended throughout the length of the weapon; movements must remain relaxed, supple and efficient while managing a weighty object; and footwork must be agile to allow rapid changes in the actual fighting range. Within the Chen style numerous weapons are practiced, including sword, broadsword, spear, *guan dao*, pole, double-sword, double-broadsword and double iron mace.

The forms are at once practical and aesthetic. Artistically pleasing to watch, the weapons routines are physically complex and demanding to complete. Many of the weapon forms have changed little since the time of Chen Wangting. Consequently they provide a window to the origins of Taijiquan and represent an important legacy to today's Taijiquan practitioner.

Sword (Jian)

The sword is one of the most ancient weapons in Chinese martial arts history. Archaeologists have discovered swords from as early as the Bronze Age. When the Terracotta Army was unearthed in the early Chinese capital Xian, a find dating back to the Qin dynasty more than two thousand years ago, the officers and generals were found carrying swords. Some of the earliest Chinese literature recounts the experience of Li Zu, a disciple of Confucius, performing sword techniques for his master.

Legend has it that Huang Di (the Yellow Emperor) gathered metal from Shou Shan (Mountain) to forge swords more than three thousand years ago. Early Chinese swords utilized hard metal, much like the solid metal weapons used in Western medieval times. In combat, cleaving and slicing techniques were favored. Generally those using larger, heavier swords, i.e., larger, stronger warriors, prevailed over their opponents. With developments in sword technology, success depended more upon skill, precision and speed. Characterized by flexible, lively and elegant movements, the sword was a weapon for gentlemen, scholars and officers. Its essence is captured in the Chinese martial arts saying: *"Dao [broadsword] like a fierce tiger, jian [sword] like a swimming dragon."*

One of the short weapons of Chen Taijiquan, the sword is usually light in weight, with a flexible blade. Unlike the broadsword, the sword has cutting edges on both sides, as well as a sharp tip for stabbing motions. At the base of the handle is a metal pommel that is used to strike backwards. The weapon is divided into sections, each having its own particular function. The first third of the blade, from the tip down, is extremely sharp, though not very strong. The middle section of the sword is a little stronger, and though not so sharp, can still be used to cut. The bottom third, closest to the guard, is much stronger with blunt edges.

The sword's flexibility enables its wielder to inflict injury from a multitude of angles using many different methods. With the great versatility of the weapon, it is said that there is *"no gap the sword cannot enter, and no gap that another can enter."*

Chen Taijiquan contains one single straight sword form consisting of forty-nine postures. The forty-nine

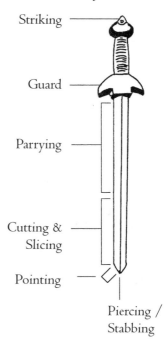

FIGURE 6.1
Diagram of a sword showing the different compoents

Striking

Guard

Parrying

Cutting &
Slicing

Pointing

Piercing /
Stabbing

postures can be sub-divided into thirteen basic techniques: *zha* (thrusting downwards); *ci* (level or upward thrust); *dian* (pointing by flicking the wrist); *pi* (chop); *mo* (slicing levelly or obliquely upwards); *sao* (sweeping); *hua* (neutralizing in a circular path); *liao* (circular deflection with point uppermost); *gua* (hang); *tuo* (push up); *tui* (push); *jie* (intercept); and *jia* (raise opponent's weapon overhead).

When performing the sword form, the practitioner must clearly understand which technique is being executed and put energy into the appropriate part of the sword. For example, when absorbing or parrying an opponent's weapon, energy should be projected to the bottom two-thirds of the edge of the sword closest to the handle. In cutting movements, energy is projected to the first third of the weapon. Thrusting and stabbing actions require the energy to be at the tip of the sword, with the weapon moving straight into the target. Pointing or pecking movements use the tip plus the first two centimeters of the sword. Given the light weight of the sword in relation to other weapons, failure to use the correct part of the weapon for a particular action could easily result in its being broken.

Weapons training is an important part of the Chen training curriculum. The various weapons each train different qualities necessary in developing a "Taijiquan physique." Practicing the Chen sword form allows an exponent to develop the ability to project energy in a relaxed manner to the tip of the sword. It also helps to create an efficient Taiji body, with repeated practice loosening the large joints such as the hips and shoulders. It can help to develop the flexibility of the wrists and hands. Using Taijiquan's comfortable, expansive body movement, practicing the sword requires agility and balanced footwork. Following the characteristics of Chen style Taijiquan, the routine should exhibit coiling and twining actions, constantly changing between fast and slow, as well as soft and hard movements. The principles of sticking, adhering and following an opponent, body leading the movement of the sword, and movement being continuous without break must all be evident.

A thorough knowledge of the barehand routine is a prerequisite if the sword form is to be performed to a high standard. The stances, methods of employing force and the movement principles of the sword form are identical to the barehanded forms. Only by building upon the foundation of the handform can the practitioner use the *yi* to lead the qi and the qi to drive the body. Without this foundation, efforts to project the body's *jing* to the sword will be futile.

Given the variety of methods with which the sword can be used, it must be held in a relaxed grip. This is necessary if the Chen Taijiquan sword practitioner is to change rapidly and freely according to the technique. Gripping the handle forcefully with the index finger inhibits the palm's ability to maneuver the position of the sword. There are several ways that the sword can be carried. The most frequently used method is holding the handle with the hand touching the guard, grasping primarily with the thumb and middle two fingers. To enable maximum flexibility when changing from one technique to another, the palm remains empty (*xu*), pressing lightly against the handle of the sword. During the course of the sword form it is occasionally necessary to execute movements more forcefully—for example, in the movement Left Side Holds Up One Thousand Pounds (*Zuo Tuo Cien Jin*). In this case, the thumb and all four fingers hold the handle tightly.

An instantly recognizable feature of the Taijiquan sword form is the way the swordsman positions his empty hand. The index and middle fingers point forward, while the end of the thumb makes a circle with the tips of the other two fingers to form the characteristic "sword fingers." Coordinating the sword fingers with the movements of the sword serves to maintain the body's equilibrium. Held in this manner, the sword fingers may also be used to attack vital areas of an opponent such as the throat or eyes.

Aesthetically pleasing to watch or perform, the sword form, not only strengthens the body but can raise the spirit of the practitioner, once mastered. In his book *The Art of Chen Family Taijiquan*, Chen Zhenglei cites a verse composed by one of his teachers, Chen Zhaopei, extolling the benefits of practicing the sword:

> *Zha* [thrusting downwards], *dian* [pointing by flicking
> the wrist], *mo* [slicing levelly or obliquely upwards],
> *pi* [chop], *ci* [level or upward thrust] draw into spirals,
> leading the attacker's energy harmlessly.
> *Tiao* [splitting from bottom to top] and
> *li* [splitting from top to bottom] is the correct way;
> *tui tuo* [push and lift up] is the orthodox method.
> There are means by which to advance while
> leading the attacker in; the horizontal and vertical movements
> of the sword a flash of steel. Contracting like a hedgehog:
> releasing energy like reaching to the end of a rainbow.
> A myriad of sun rays radiates brilliantly;
> the glorious radiance is marvellously boundless.

After long practice with the Taiji sword;
at the time your skill is perfected,
you will achieve an enlightenment of your own.

Chen Taijiquan Straight Sword

1. Preparation Form

2. Homage to the Sun

3. Immortal Points the Way

4. Blue Dragon Out of the Water

5. Protect the Knees

6. Closing the Door

7. Blue Dragon Out of the Water

8. Turn and Chop Down

9. Blue Dragon Turns Over

10. Flying Diagonally

11. Spread Wings

12. Nod the Head

13. Separate Grass to Seek Snake

14. Golden Rooster Stands Alone

15. Immortal Points the Way

16. Cover and Block

17. Ancient Tree Wraps Its Roots

18. Hungry Tiger Attacks for Food

19. Blue Dragon Sways Its Tail

20. Turning the Arm Backward

21. Wild Horse Leaps the Ravine

22. White Snake Shows Its Tongue

23. Black Dragon Sways Its Tail

24. Zhong Kui Holds the Sword

25. Louhan Subdues Dragon

26. Black Bear Turns Backward

27. Swallow Pecks the Mud

28. White Snake Shows Its Tongue

29. Flying Diagonally

30. Eagle and Bear Battle with their Wits

31. Swallow Pecks the Mud

32. Pluck Stars and Change the Constellations

33. Scoop Moon from Under Sea

34. Phoenix Nods Its Head

35. Swallow Pecks the Mud

36. White Snake Shows Its Tongue

37. Flying Diagonally

38. Left Side Holds Up One Thousand Pounds

39. Right Side Holds Up One Thousand Pounds

40. Swallow Pecks the Mud

41. White Ape Offering Fruit

42. Falling Flowers

43. Jab Upward then Downward

44. Flying Diagonally

45. Na Dra Explores the Sea

46. The Large Serpent Turns Itself Around

47. Wei Tor Presents Pestle

48. Millstone Turning Sword

49. Return to Taiji

Broadsword (Dao)

Introduced to China as a result of the Mongol invasions, the broadsword with its characteristic curved blade became the most widely used short weapon in military circles. Its popularity was such that it eclipsed the older straight sword (jian) as the dominant military sidearm after the fifteenth century.

One of the short weapon forms of Chen Taijiquan, the broadsword form encompassed just thirteen movements prior to the 1930s. Between 1930 and 1938, eighteenth-generation Chen style master Chen Zhaopei taught Taijiquan at the famous Nanjing Central Kuoshu Institute. Feeling that the form was too short, he added an additional nine movements, creating the form practiced in Chenjiagou today. Even with the extra movements, the Chen Taijiquan Single Broadsword form is a very short and dynamic routine. In character, this weapon is often likened to a fierce tiger, with each movement being more direct and obvious than the straight sword.

Although a short weapon, the broadsword can cover a deceptively long distance through the use of explosive leaping and jumping. Movements can be performed differently depending upon the goal of practice. Often the form is executed with long, low stances as a means of conditioning the body, increasing one's power and speed. Very low stances, however, lack the nimbleness necessary for

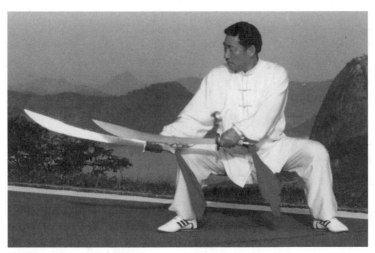

FIGURE 6.2 Chen Xiaowang demonstrating Double Broadsword

combat use. When focusing on the applications of the broadsword, emphasis should be on higher postures to increase mobility. To acquire both martial and conditioning benefits, the practitioner should train over a range of heights.

In contrast to the sword, which is double-edged and light, the broadsword is single-edged and heavy. The strength of the weapon means that cutting movements tend to be large, expansive and powerful. In appearance, using the broadsword is *"like splitting a mountain."* Like the other weapons of the Chen style, it is important that the broadsword be practiced only after a good foundation has been attained through the barehanded boxing routines.

When performing the broadsword routine, the practitioner alternates between the body leading the broadsword and the broadsword leading the body. Techniques must be precise, clearly fulfilling the application requirements. Traditionally the weapon has thirteen different techniques attributed to it: *gun* (parrying by turning to the left); *bi* (parrying by closing to the right); *zha* (thrust); *lan* (deflecting with the rear side of the broadsword); *pi* (chopping vertically); *kan* (cutting); *liao* (circular deflection with point facing upwards); *jie* (blocking with the edge); *chan* (circular twisting); *dou* (shaking); *jia* (raising opponent's weapon overhead); *mo* (slicing either levelly or diagonally upwards); and *tiao* (upward flicking motion using the top of the weapon).

In practice the whole body moves together, with the waist as the axis. The practitioner must coil the broadsword closely around the head and body. This follows the broadsword technique of *"chan tou dao"* or *"circling-around-the-head knife,"* where the blunt edge of the weapon is reeled around the head and body to divert an opponent's weapon or to attack.

Within Chinese martial arts circles there is a saying that *"to know the single broadsword follow the left hand."* Throughout the routine, equal attention should be given to the empty hand and how it is used to regulate the weapon's movements. At times, the hand is used for blocking or clearing. Sometimes the empty palm supports the blunt edge of the weapon, adding strength to the technique. The empty hand can also act to counterbalance actions of the broadsword.

Chen Taijiquan Broadsword Form

1. Preparation Form

2. Protect the Heart

3. Green Dragon Out of the Water

4. Wind Blows the Flowers

5. White Cloud Covers Roof

6. Black Tiger Searching the Mountain

7. Shu Qin Carries the Sword on His Back

8. Golden Rooster Stands on One Leg

9. Rolling Away from the Wind

10. Cut White Snake Body

11. Three Rings Around the Sun

12. Move the Clouds to See the Sun

13. Beat Grass to Find Snake Left

14. Beat Grass to Find Snake Right

15. Green Dragon Out of the Water

16. Wind Blows the Flowers

17. Wild Goose Opens Wings

18. Ye Cha Searches the Ocean

19. Left Turning the Body to Cut

20. Right Turning the Body to Cut

21. White Snake Spits Tongue

22. Holding the Moon

23. Closing Form

Spear (Qiang)

Also referred to as the "Pear-Flower Spear and White Ape Staff" (*Li Hua Qiang Jia Bai Yuan Kun*), the Chen Taijiquan spear is practiced with a form containing the functions of both spear and staff. Chen Wangting is credited with formulating the routine, making it one of the most ancient Taiji forms. In his comprehensive review of Taijiquan, *The Origin, Evolution and Development of Shadow Boxing*, Gu Liuxin refers to the evidence of historian Tang Hao, who concluded that Chen Wangting was greatly influenced by the writings of Ming general Qi Jiguang when formulating his own family system of boxing. Qi Jiguang, in turn, greatly admired the spear techniques of the Yang Family 24-Spear Form, including it in his military training text. The Yang family referred to should not be confused with the Yang family responsible for propagating Yang style Taijiquan. Instead, it refers to a famous female warrior of the Song dynasty who used the 24-movement spear form when avenging the deaths of all her male relatives.

In creating the original version of the Chen Taiji spear form, Chen Wangting followed the pattern of the Yang 24-movement form in posture and name. The uniqueness of his form came through applying Taiji movement principles to the existing techniques. Since the time of Chen Wangting, the Chen spear form has grown from 24 to 72 movements with the addition of a variety of staff movements.

When the routine is performed well, the martial roots of the spear form become obvious. Few movements are done slowly. The overall tempo is forceful, direct and rapid, with an unpredictability likened to thunder and lightning. Utilizing numerous explosive releases of power or *fajing*, the form takes just two minutes or so to complete, despite its length. Within Chinese *wushu* circles, the spear is considered to be an advanced weapon. This is reflected in it being recognized as the "King of Weapons."

To correctly execute the movements of the spear form, the practitioner should be well versed in the postural requirements and

FIGURE 6.3
Chen Zhenglei teaching the spear form in Chenjiagou

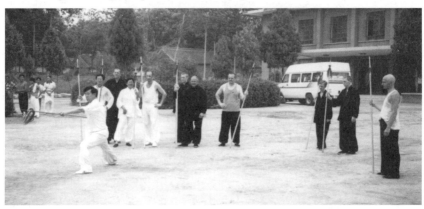

footwork methods of the handforms. Through prolonged practice of the basic forms and exercises, sufficient upper-body strength and overall flexibility must be developed to meet the high demands of the spear form. As well as being aesthetically pleasing, the Chen family spear form is a highly practical training tool. While the practitioner is unlikely to meet with an occasion requiring him to use this weapon in combat, spear practice will enhance barehand skills by improving balance through the use of intricate and rapid stepping movements.

The spear form and the practice of individual movements with the spear can help to develop stronger energy more rapidly. This is especially true for the energy that is transmitted from the back and through the shoulders and arms. When executing the form, close consideration must be paid to the coordination of the eyes, hands, stances and stepping. A widely quoted expression—*"one hundred days to practice broadsword, one thousand days to practice spear"*—reflects the intricacy and level of difficulty inherent in the form.

Applications can switch instantly from spear to staff techniques. Watching the form, one sees a clear distinction between the two. In the thrusting actions of the Pear-Flower Spear, the head of the weapon is used in predominantly piercing movements. This is contrasted with the hitting movements of the White Ape Staff, where the shaft of the spear is utilized to strike, block or deflect. In common with the other weapons of the Chen style, the concepts of sticking and listening are applied when practicing spear.

Chen Taijiquan Pear-Flower Spear and White Ape Staff

1. Ye Cha (Night Ghost) Explores the Sea Bottom

2. Cutting Whole Circle

3. Middle Level Thrust

4. Three Swift Thrusts

5. High Level Thrust

6. Swaying Pearl-Beaded Curtain

7. Lower Level Thrust

8. Turn Around and Thrust

9. The Black Dragon Presents Claws

10. Step Forward with One Thrust

11. Sweep the Floor to Thrust

12. Side Block

13. Throw Two Forward Hits

14. Yellow Dragon Manipulates the Shaft

15. Down-to-Up Strike

16. Turn Around to Make One Half Circle

17. Blocking Thrust at Waist Level

18. Make One Half Circle

19. Spear Touches Ground Like a Snake

20. Suddenly Lift the Spear

21. Deliver a Thrust

22. Two Covering Thrusts

23. Wave Banner from Left Side

24. Thrusting Toward the Sky

25. Raise Flag to Sweep on Right Side

26. The Iron Ox Ploughs

27. Turn Around to Make One Half Circle

28. Thrust Like Dripping Water

29. Two Covering Thrusts

30. Mount Dragon and Deliver Rapid Thrust

31. Parting Grass to Look for Snake

32. The White Ape Drags Spear

33. The Black Dragon Returns to the Den

34. Taking Back the Pipa

35. Throw Two Forward Hits

36. Wield Banner to Sweep Ground

37. Mount Tai Crushes Egg

38. Turn Around to Make One Half Circle

39. Cat Catches Mouse

40. Thrust from the Left

41. Thrust from the Right

42. Turn Around to Deliver Thrust

43. Prop Up Heel

44. One-Arm Thrust

45. Cutting Whole Circle

46. Second Son Carries the Mountain and Sweeping Thrust

47. Cut One Half Circle

48. Lower Parting Thrust

49. Turn Around to Make One Half Circle

50. Falcon Diving into Quail Flock

51. Sweeping Thrust from Left

52. Lifting Heel

53. One Thrust

54. Cutting Whole Circle

55. Second Son Carries the Mountain and Sweeping Thrust

56. Cut One Half Circle

57. Fair Lady Threads Needle

58. Jade Lady Works Shuttles

59. Assassination Thrust

60. Turn Around to Sweep Thrust

61. Cutting Whole Circle

62. Protect the Knees

63. Two Covering Thrusts

64. Black Dragon Sways Its Tail

65. Block Once Forward

66. Block Forward Again

67. Block from Left

68. Block from Right

69. Cut One Half Circle

70. Old Man Fishing

71. Turn Around to Deliver Thrust

72. Finish

Spring and Autumn Broadsword (Guan Dao)

Variously known as the "Spring and Autumn Broadsword," the "Green Dragon Crescent Moon Broadsword" or simply the "Big

Knife," the *guan dao* was the favored weapon of the renowned General Guan Yu. During the turbulent Three Kingdoms Period (A.D. 25–220) of Chinese history, he was famous for his great strength, martial ability and readiness to champion the cause of the oppressed. Eventually deified and given the title of "Military Sage," Guan Yu is usually portrayed in paintings or statues with a long beard, red face and stern expression. Invariably he is pictured carrying his favorite long-handled, double-edged broadsword.

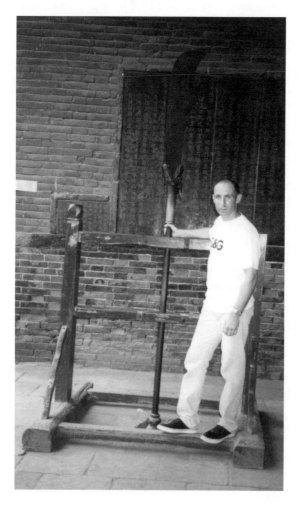

FIGURE 6.3
David Gaffney at Guan Yu's temple with the replica of General Guan's famous weapon

Also the preferred weapon of Chen Wangting, the *guan dao* is one of the oldest weapon forms in the system. Characterized by strong and powerful movements, the *guan dao* is a large and heavy weapon. To the observer the form should give off a spirit of expansiveness and ferocity.

The high physical demands of this weapon necessitate a thorough grounding in the core skills of Chen Taijiquan. To manipulate the weapon fluidly and in a relaxed manner requires a stable root and a high degree of upper-body strength. Chen Taijiquan *guan dao* teaches the practitioner to move and be aware in any direction. The form can be divided into thirteen fundamental techniques, each of which must be expressed clearly in the form. These are: *pi* (cleave or chop vertically); *kan* (cut horizontally); *liao* (circular slice upwards); *gua* (hang); *zhan* (circular cut); *mo* (level slice); *tui* (push); *zhi* (pierce); *lan* (intercept); *jia* (raise opponent's weapon overhead); *tuo* (draw); *tiao* (lift upwards with the end of the blade); and *zhai* (forward parry).

While the individual names of the weapon or hand forms describe the movements, the *guan dao* form is unique. Each of the thirty movements of this form is given a seven-character song or poem. When taken together, they relate the story of General Guan. So each time the form is practiced, his exploits are re-enacted.

The mastery of Chen Wangting with this weapon, combined with the fact that he also had a long beard, led him to acquire the nickname "Equal to Guan Yu." His exploits with the *guan dao* are mentioned in the *Genealogy of the Chen Family*, where it is recorded that:

Wangting, alias Zhouting, was a knight at the end of the Ming dynasty and a scholar in the early years of the Qing Dynasty. He was known in Shandong Province as a master of martial arts, once defeating more than a thousand bandits. He was the originator of the barehanded and armed combat boxing of the Chen school. He was a born warrior, as can be proved by the broadsword he used in combat.

Chen Taijiquan *Guan Dao*

1. General Guan Carries Broadsword
2. Clouds Over the Head
3. Holding the Moon
4. Three Upward Movements
5. Three Downward Movements
6. White Ape Draws the Broadsword
7. Entire Circular Movement
8. Tiger Leaps Suddenly
9. Parting Mane
10. Cross Broadsword
11. Turning Waist and Twisting Root
12. Circulate and Strike Upward
13. Holding the Moon
14. Circulate and Strike Downward
15. Holding the Moon
16. Entire Circular Movement Twist Body Strike
17. Backward Strike
18. Circulate and Strike Down
19. Clouds Over the Head
20. Circulate and Strike Upward
21. Lift Up Green Dragon
22. Circulate and Strike Downward

23. Clouds Over the Head

24. Offer Wine, Pick Up Cloak, Suddenly Turning Back

25. Bronze Gavel

26. Double Kick

27. Iron Bar

28. Rolling Curtain

29. Crossing Strike

30. Dragon Wades in the Water

The Chen weapon forms are tangible links to the martial past of China. Preserved and passed down through the generations, they speak loudly about what Taijiquan must have been like centuries ago.

CHAPTER SEVEN

Chen Family Legends

History in China is like an old man's memory. The distant past is often more vivid than the present. The stories are often dramatized and exaggerated by frequent telling.

The Chinese have always looked to their ancestors for direction and their sense of duty in life. Their history is full of moral examples to be drawn on and evaluated anew in every generation. History to the Chinese is not an objective account of the past but morality tales in which heroes and villains are made relevant in the present day.

A Pair of Heroes Defeat the Bandits

The village of Beipingao in Wen County (Wenxian) is famous for the beauty of its bamboo forest. At the time of the events that are about to unfold, the population of several thousand enjoyed a certain degree of wealth and prosperity and lived contentedly.

It was just before the lunar New Year, when all the families were gathered in preparation for the festivities. Unnoticed by the residents, a group of bandits slipped into the village, led by two brothers who were particularly repulsive in appearance. They were "Flying Centipede" (*Li Jiang*) and "Poison Scorpion" (*Li Her*). As soon as they entered, the leaders commanded their men to seal off the village, guarding strategic vantage points to ensure that nobody could leave or enter. The brothers ordered the villagers to hand over all their valuables, and also to gather all their presentable maidens so they could be selected as the wives of the bandits. The villagers were informed that the punishment for anyone defying these orders would be the execution of their entire family.

During the quiet of the night, all the village elders and the menfolk, led by a man named Wang, held a meeting to find a solution to their predicament. However, despite much discussion, they could arrive at no practical solution. Just as all started to despair, a young woman who had been present to serve the menfolk tea stepped forward, stating that she might have an answer. She had recently married into the village from the nearby village of Chenjiagou. At this time, a woman's view would rarely have been solicited, but because of the urgency of the situation, she was encouraged to speak.

The woman, whose surname was Chen, informed those gathered that her family had a long history of martial arts, starting from the first-generation descendant Chen Bu. The present ninth-generation leader Chen Wangting, having devised the new art of Taijiquan, had incited a new wave of enthusiasm for martial arts in the village. Most of the young men in Chenjiagou practiced martial arts, and even the women were taught. With this, the young woman suggested that help should be sought from her home village. When no one was brave enough or strong enough to offer to fight through the bandits guarding the village, the young woman volunteered. Armed with a sword, she killed the two bandits guarding the eastern aspect of the village with ease and sped through the winter night until she arrived at the home of her father, Chen Soule.

Chen Soule was of the tenth generation of the Chen clan, a nephew of Chen Wangting. He was taught by Chen Wangting and was highly skilled in the family system. Besides the daughter who now lived in Beipingao, he had twin sons who, at the time of the story, were about sixteen years of age. They were Chen Shenru and Chen Xunru, nicknamed "Big Sky God" and "Little Sky God."

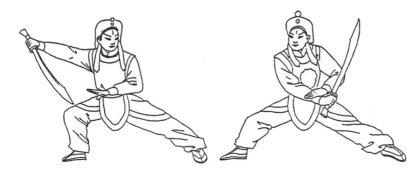

FIGURE 7.1 Drawing of pair of heroes

Both were already proficient in the martial arts, having been taught by their father and supervised by Chen Wangting.

Upon hearing about the plight of Beipingao, the two young brothers volunteered to return with their sister to rid the village of the brigands. After consulting with Chen Wangting and getting his endorsement, the three siblings set off. That evening, the brothers surprised the bandits, as they were not expecting any resistance. The twins were heavily outnumbered, but nevertheless dealt with the bandits in one fell swoop. The two bandit leaders were defeated and slain.

To celebrate their heroism, the husband of the young woman composed a drama based on the events titled "A Pair of Heroes Defeat the Bandits" *(Shuan Yin Puo Di)*. For many years afterwards it was performed during village festivals.

The incident is significant in that it marked the "coming out" of Taijiquan, when the skill devised by Chen Wangting was first used in combat. Those who had mocked and doubted the practicalities of the art began to change their views.

Chenjiagou Taijiquan Will Not Be Taught to the Female Line

Chen Xunru of the eleventh generation of the Chen family lineage is remembered as the person who decreed that the family art be taught only to male descendants and not to females.

Members of the female line of the Chen family had, up until this time, distinguished themselves in combat many times. When Chen Xunru and his twin brother Chen Shenru rescued the villagers of Beipingao, their sister battled with great courage and skill during fierce fighting against the troublesome bandits, ably assisting them. Their father Chen Soule had a sister, Chen Souyu, who was highly skilled in martial arts and once saved the life of her brother when he was in mortal danger while dealing with an enemy.

When Chen Shenru and Chen Xunru were eighteen years old, they were found wives from good families. In time, a daughter was born to Chen Shenru, and two sons to Chen Xunru. When the

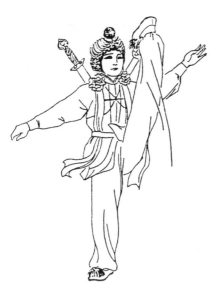

daughter of Chen Shenru, Chen Ziaoniu, was only a year old, her father fell ill one day after a training session, dying six months later. Chen Xunru adopted his twin's daughter and taught her alongside his own sons. Ziaoniu excelled in the family martial system, surpassing the young men of the family in skill.

Time passed and Chen Ziaoniu came of marriageable age, when an incident occurred that was to affect the women of Chenjiagou for many years.

FIGURE 7.2 Drawing of female warrior

Rejecting a young man's proposal of marriage, the Chen family inadvertently offended his wealthy family and set in motion a tragic sequence of events. The young man's rejection was compounded when an honest young man named Zhao was chosen for her. The wealthy family's son, Zhang Wai, who possessed some martial skill, began to threaten and harass the Zhao family, damaging property and crops, as well as injuring members of the family. After enduring many months of such treatment, Ziaoniu's patience finally gave way when old man Zhao, her father-in-law, was attacked. Ignoring a promise she had made to Chen Xunru not to show her martial ability to her new family, she dealt with the bully and his bodyguards with ease.

Ziaoniu's husband, although honest, was nevertheless a timid and cowardly man. Rather than showing gratitude to his wife, he instead blamed her for being the source of his family's troubles. When old man Zhao subsequently died from the injuries inflicted on him, young Zhao, in a supreme act of cowardice, sought to settle the issue with Zhang Wai by denouncing his wife and sending her back to her family. At the time this was considered to be the greatest shame and dishonor that could befall a woman. In despair, Ziaoniu broke the sword given to her by her family and vowed never to practice martial arts again. Grief-stricken, she eventually hung herself and was buried with her broken sword. Chen Xunru vowed that from this day forward, the female members of the family in Chenjiagou were not to be taught Taijiquan.

Chen Jingbo's Fight to the Death with "Black Tiger"

Chen Jingbo, also known as Chen Changqin, belonged to the twelfth generation of the Chen family. Taught Taijiquan by Chen Zhengru, the brother of the famous twins Shenru and Xunru, he excelled in all the family weapons, and his martial arts skill was of the highest level. A famous incident is often recounted about his service as a policeman in Shandong Province.

Stealing a horse from the official stable, a notorious thief left a note challenging anyone to come after him. No one was brave enough to give chase, as he was known to be a formidable fighter. Chen Jingbo, however, on hearing of the incident was undeterred and accepted the challenge. Eventually meeting up with the thief,

Chen Jingbo offered a challenge of his own. He suggested that the thief attack him three times while he (Chen) kept his hands behind his back. Agreeing that if defeated he would return with Chen Jingbo, the thief pulled out a broadsword and thrust it towards Chen's throat. Very calmly but with great speed, Chen ducked slightly and caught the tip of the broadsword in his teeth. No matter how hard the thief tried to draw it back, he was unable to do so. With a turn of the neck, Chen deflected the force to one side, throwing the thief down onto the ground. This famous story was written in many books in China.

Chen Jingbo later became an armed escort and travelled in the provinces for several years. His reputation was such that bandits were afraid to attack the goods that he was defending. In his last engagement before retiring to Chenjiagou, he came across a man called Wang Dingguo or "Black Tiger." Black Tiger, although possessing some martial skill, was not a man of good character. Often he would demand money from the villagers and beat anyone who dared to defy him. On this particular day he was demonstrating his skill in the courtyard of a temple in order to intimidate the people. Vigorously demonstrating both barehand and weapons forms, Black Tiger was just about to demonstrate a broadsword routine when Chen Jingbo arrived. Boasting loudly that if anyone could throw a bowl of water on him as he performed the routine he would quietly leave the area, Black Tiger dared anyone in the crowd to take up his challenge. At this point, Chen Jingbo stepped forward. Black Tiger, on seeing an older man, asked for a bowl of water to be brought.

The demonstration then began. As the broadsword spun around, Chen was able to spot a gap. Before anyone could see what had happened, Black Tiger stood there with the bowl on his head, water dripping down his face. In Chen's hand was the cap that Black Tiger had been wearing a few moments before. Filled with shame and utterly humiliated, Black Tiger inquired after Chen's name and home village and angrily retorted that he would seek Chen out one day.

Chen Jingbo retired from escort service and returned to Chenjiagou. He took up farming and teaching the younger generation in the village. He also continued to exchange skills with his contemporaries, particularly Chen Jixia. During this period the two were famous for their excellence, Chen Jingbo specializing in *kao* (body strike) and Chen Jixia specializing in *zhou* (elbow strike).

On a summer's day, in a rare mood, both men decided to perform sword sparring. As the younger generation had never witnessed such an event, there was great excitement in the village. After about thirty techniques, Chen Jingbo, who was over seventy years of age, became tired and decided to stop. That same evening he became ill and collapsed in his home. Recovery was slow and Chen Jingbo had to rest his body. Finally, as autumn approached, he was well enough to ride his donkey into Wenxian for market day.

While Chen Jingbo was away, a monk arrived at Chenjiagou inquiring after his whereabouts. On hearing that Chen was in Wenxian, he made his way there. Chen, riding his donkey home, decided to take a rest in a broken temple. It was here that he met the monk, who was none other than Black Tiger. Chen wanted to avoid a fight, as he was still recovering from his illness; however, Black Tiger was happy to find a weakened Chen. Since their last meeting, Black Tiger had improved his martial skill by returning to his teacher, who happened to be a brother of Flying Centipede and Poison Scorpion, the two brothers killed by the Chen twins in Beipinguo. Still vividly remembering his own humiliation and urged on by his teacher, Black Tiger's mind was doubly filled with vengeance.

Chen Jingbo realized that a fight was inevitable, and that the Chen family's honor was at stake. With this, they began fighting.

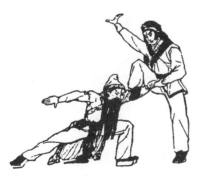

FIGURE 7.3 Drawing depicting fight of Chen Jingbo and Black Tiger

After a prolonged engagement, Chen used his famous body strike to send Black Tiger crashing into the stone wall of the temple, cracking his head open and killing him outright. Chen Jingbo himself collapsed with exhaustion. He was taken back to Chenjiagou where he died a few days later. Many stories were written about the "fight to the death with Wang Dingguo."

A One-Eyed Master Fights at the Teahouse

Chen Yao was of the sixteenth generation of the Chen family, the eldest son of Chen Zhongsheng and elder brother of Chen Xin.

The incident in question happened at a popular roadside teahouse. One day a group of policemen arrived at the teahouse. From their demeanor, it was immediately obvious that they were in bad humor. Cursing at anyone who happened to be in their way, and threateningly making loud clanging noises with their various weapons (broadswords and iron maces among others), they caused most of the other customers to quickly leave for fear of trouble. Once seated, they complained vociferously that the tea served to them was too hot to drink and ordered the waiter to take the bowls outside to the courtyard so that the breeze could cool them down.

At this moment a group of farmers arrived at the teahouse. It was midday on a hot summer's day, and all the workers were hot and thirsty. The owner of the teahouse kept a large urn outside in the courtyard, where he would collect the leftover tea from customers' teapots. Periodically he would add some water so that the urn was kept full. Workers from the surrounding area were able to quench their thirst from the urn without charge. A piece of wood was placed across the urn, on which were placed some old drinking bowls.

On this particular day one of the farm workers, who happened to be new to the area, mistakenly picked up one of the bowls of tea that was cooling for the policemen on the table next to the urn. Thirstily drinking the tea, he loudly declared how good it was.

With this he picked up another bowl of tea and handed it to an old man sitting under a tree. When the policemen demanded their tea and found that they were two bowls short, they cursed loudly, threatening to beat up the waiter.

Hearing the commotion, the old man under the tree stood up. Unremarkable to look at, he was a small, thin, man blind in one eye. He politely apologized for the mistake; however, the policemen were not satisfied. Hurling insults at the old man, one of them picked up a bowl of hot tea and flung it at him. Before anyone could see what happened, the old man turned his body to the side, avoiding the bowl, and before the bowl fell to the ground, crouched and caught it in his hand. Not a drop of tea landed on him. In a rage, the senior policeman drew his broadsword and chopped towards the old man. Three successive chops were all easily evaded. His patience understandably wearing thin, the old man warned the policeman to stop while he could. Unable to recognize superior martial skill, the policeman darted forward again with the broadsword. After side-stepping nine such charges, the old man with lightning speed grabbed the sword-wielding hand in a tight vice-like grip and by twisting, he dislodged the weapon. Overcome with pain, the policeman felt as if all the tendons in his wrist had been torn. Seeing their leader's defeat, all of his friends surged forwards in a combined attack. However, they were no match for the old man. With nimble footwork and rapid techniques he felled them all. Those who received his *zhou* (elbow) and *kao* (body strike) techniques were badly hurt. Without waiting for the consequences, the old man left.

This is the story of how Chen Yao defeated the policemen at the teahouse.

Chen Xin's Heart and Blood

Chen Xin, also called Pinsan, was of the sixteenth generation of the Chen family. His father Chen Zhongsheng and uncle Chen

Jishen were twins, and both were very skilled Taijiquan practitioners. Passing the military examination at the same time, both
became *Wuxiang* (fifth-degree ranking officers). Chen Zhongsheng
was famous for using a thirty-pound iron spear on the battlefield.
Chen Xin and his elder brother Chen Yao were taught by their
father, a middle son having died at an early age.

Within Chenjiagou a family tradition existed at that time with
regard to the birth of any male offspring. When the child was one
hundred days old, he would be brought before a table upon which
were placed three items—a knife, a writing brush and money.
Whichever the child picked would determine his future. The three
items symbolized whether one was to learn martial arts, study literature or go into commerce. Although this was not absolute, families used this test widely as an indication for the future path in life
a child should pursue. It is said that Chen Yao picked up a knife,
and Chen Xin picked up a writing brush. Chen Zhongsheng was
happy for one son to follow a martial career, and one to follow a
literary path.

Chen Xin, however, was greatly inspired by the martial skill he
witnessed around him, and although asked to concentrate on literature, paid careful attention to the martial practice and teaching
around him. After his father died, he concentrated all his efforts
into improving his Taijiquan. Although never attaining the level of
his elder brother, Chen Xin was nevertheless a very good Taiji
practitioner in his own right. Realizing that there was a lack of
written instructions on the family art, as teaching had always been
in the form of oral transmission, he became concerned that some
skill might be lost in each successive generation. With this, he
made a firm decision to write and expound the principles and
methods of Chen Family Taijiquan. His most famous book is
Illustrated Explanation of Chen Family Taijiquan (Chen Shi Taijiquan Tushuo).
The book took him twelve years to write, from the thirty-fourth
year of Emperor Guangxu (1908) until the eighth-year of the
Republic (1919). Written entirely by hand, the teachings of many
generations of Chen family Taijiquan masters were explained in

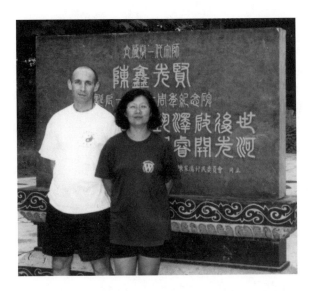

FIGURE 7.4
The authors at Chen
Xin's memorial stone in
front of the Chen
Village Training Hall

detail, with numerous illustrations, without keeping anything secret. It is the most systematic and complete work on Chen style Taijiquan.

During the period when he was writing the book, the region experienced many natural disasters, leading to an exodus of the able-bodied from the village. Life was extremely hard. Chen Xin was in his seventies and in poor health. He amended and rewrote the book four times before he was completely satisfied. By the time the final manuscript was completed, he was very ill. In the eighteenth year of the Republic (1929), he sent for his nephew, Chen Chunyun, who was in Hunan Province, as he had no children of his own. The nephew returned to find his uncle lying in bed. Chen Xin handed him the manuscript and said, "This is the result of my heart and blood *(xin xue)*. Transmit it to those who deserve it, otherwise burn it. Be sure not to give it to arrogant or ignorant people." He died that same night.

Because of the abject poverty, Chen Chunyun was unable to give his uncle a proper burial. In the twenty-first year of the Republic (1932), Tang Hao, the martial arts historian, arrived at Chenjiagou while conducting his research on the history and origins of Taijiquan. He greatly appreciated being shown the manuscripts of Chen Xin. The manuscripts were eventually published in 1933 by the combined effort of the Henan Province Martial Arts Academy, the Archives Bureau and the Provincial Museum. Chen Xin was eventually laid to rest in a proper burial ceremony nearly four years after he died.

Chen Fa-ke Defeats the Red Spear Gang

Tales of human conflict preserve the memories of many famous martial artists. While each is remembered for his or her high level of fighting skill, some are also noted for their compassion and virtuousness. Chen Fa-ke (1887–1957), also known as Fusheng, was a seventeenth-generation descendant of the Chen clan. The son of the renowned Chen Yanxi and grandson of Chen Changxing, he was highly respected within the Taijiquan circles of the day, both for his martial accomplishments and for his virtuous character.

At the time of the boy's birth, Chen Fa-ke's father had already reached a mature age. Chen Fa-Ke was the sole surviving son in the family, his brothers having died in an epidemic. Being the only male child, he was somewhat spoiled and indulged during his early years. Fond of food, he tended to overeat, resulting in recurrent digestive problems. Although taught Taijiquan from a young age, Chen Fake was not serious in his practice, and it was a case of "fishing (casting out the net) for three days, drying the net for two days." Even at the age of fourteen he was still not proficient, much to the despair of his father and the disappointment of the village elders.

His attitude changed dramatically upon overhearing a conversation among the older generation at his home about the passing of his family's martial heritage. The elders spoke of Chen Fa-ke's own family line, citing his father and famous masters from the preceding generations; they discussed how each generation of this particular line had produced outstanding martial artists and upright characters. They sighed at the misfortune of seeing the line end with a "hopeless case." As a result of Chen Fa-ke's frailty and weakness, the family's tradition was sure to be lost with his generation.

Chen Fa-ke was filled with shame. He recalled how his father was noted as the martial arts instructor of the household of Yuan Shikai (first President of the Chinese Republic), how his grandfather Chen Gengyun was commemorated in Shandong for his heroic deeds in the province, and how his great-grandfather Chen Changxing, nicknamed "Mr. Ancestral Tablet" for his upright posture and reverent attitude, synthesized the family martial arts into the forms known today. Chen Fa-ke was fourteen years of age, and he had not accomplished anything.

Chen Fa-ke vowed not to let the family heritage be lost at his hands. Vowing from that day forwards to change his ways and do justice to his forebears, he resolved to practice harder than anybody else in order to make up for the wasted years. It is said that during his young days Chen Fa-ke would repeat his forms at least thirty times a day and would sometimes perform up to one hundred repetitions. Such was his determination; he maintained this schedule in all weather, whatever the season.

In three years, Chen Fa-ke raised his level of skill beyond recognition. Chen Fa-ke's cousin Chen Boqu had always been able to defeat him in pushing hands. Chen Fa-ke's progress was so remarkable that Chen Boqu believed he must have some special secret training method. He determined to uncover the secret and, for ten days, quietly climbed the wall of Chen Fa-ke's house to spy on him practicing in the courtyard. Each day Chen Fa-ke entered the courtyard with a basket filled with steamed bread. He then proceeded to practice his form thirty or so times, in between each form eating some of the bread. By the time he had finished practicing, all the bread would be gone. Chen Boqu finally understood that there were no special secrets. Chen Fa-ke's high level of skill was a reflection of his diligent efforts.

Many dramatic tales have been passed down about the exploits

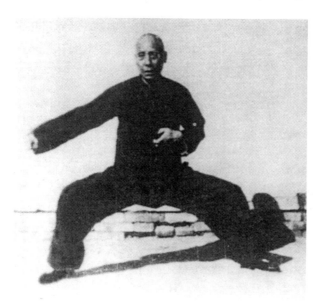

FIGURE 7.5
Chen Fa-ke in
'Green Dragon out of
the Water'

of Chen Fa-ke. One such story tells of how he helped to defend his home county, Wenxian, from bandits. During the 1920s, China was undergoing a period of political upheaval. Regions were subjugated by different warlords, and bandits roamed widely, preying on the common people. During this period Chen Fa-ke and his nephew Chen Zhaopei, five years his junior, were engaged as instructors at the Wenxian County martial arts school.

The incident began when they apprehended three robbers and handed them in to the authorities. In response, the group to which the robbers belonged kidnapped three friends of the two Chens and demanded an exchange of prisoners at a particular inn. When the Chens arrived at the inn, Chen Fa-ke asked Chen Zhaopei to stand guard outside in case there was an ambush, and he entered the inn alone to negotiate. The head of the bandits sat at a table with a gun within easy reach. Looking around, Chen Fa-ke saw the three hostages tied up on one side of the room. Chen calmly lit a cigarette, and then with lightning speed flicked the matchstick to distract the bandit. In the ensuing confusion, he managed to grab the bandit's hand as he tried to pick up the gun and followed the momentum with a hard elbow strike, breaking the man's arm. Thus the bandit leader was overcome and the hostages freed.

The incident, however, had not reached its conclusion. The next day the bandits, who were known as the "Red Spear Gang," surrounded Wenxian, threatening to seize the area. A malevolent religious sect, its members believed that they could render themselves magically invulnerable to bullets or knives. With the town in serious danger from the bandits, the Wenxian district officials asked Chen Fa-ke to lead his students to help defend the area.

Chen Fa-ke waited on the bridge leading into the city armed only with a long pole cut from a bailagan tree. Upon seeing him, one of the leaders of the bandit group charged forward in an attempt to stab him with a spear. Chen Fa-ke cried, "Let's see how impervious you are to this!" The attack was instantly parried with the wooden pole. In one fluid motion, the bandit leader's spear was dislodged from his hands, and Chen Fa-ke darted forward, piercing his opponent's body. The sight of their leader being killed so suddenly greatly unnerved the rest of the bandit group, and they immediately fled the area. Thus Chen Fa-ke saved the town from the Red Spear Gang.

Chen Zhaopei Restores the Family Treasure

Chen Zhaopei, also known as Ji Fu, belonged to the eighteenth generation of the Chen family. Born in the nineteenth year of the Emperor Guangxu, he was the son of Chen Dengke and grandson of Chen Yannien.

Chen Zhaopei nearly did not survive his infancy because his mother was unable to feed him breast milk. Suffering from malnutrition, he was in a desperately weakened condition and finally appeared to have succumbed, losing consciousness. When his family found him, his breathing was barely noticeable and they thought he had died. Rolling him in a straw mat, they left him by the river for burial. Fortunately he was discovered by villagers who heard his cries and brought him back to his family.

Despite constant treatment, Chen Zhaopei remained weak and was still not able to walk at the age of three. By the age of eight, although somewhat recovered, he still required daily medication, earning him the nickname of "Medicine jar." Out of desperation and failure to see an alternative, his father Chen Dengke decided to teach him the family art of Taijiquan. Under strict supervision and meticulous teaching for the next five years, the boy gradually became stronger and no longer needed his "medicine jar." After the death of his father, Chen Zhaopei continued to study Taijiquan from his grand-uncle Chen Yanxi, Chen Xin and his uncle Chen Fa-ke.

By the age of eighteen, Chen Zhaopei's Taiji skills were so accomplished that he was praised by the family elders. In his twenties, because of poverty, he decided to leave the village and make a career in business in order to support his mother. During this period he never failed to practice Taiji every day, no matter how busy or tired he was. It was during one such practice session, while staying at an inn, that he was spotted and thus began his lifetime of teaching Taijiquan.

With the fall of the Qing dynasty (1927) and the establishment of the Republic, China was in turmoil, with many uprisings. Worried for the safety of his aged mother, Chen Zhaopei decided to return to Chenjiagou. During this time Wenxian and its surrounding areas were overrun by bandits and robbers who looted and pillaged at will, causing great anxiety among the people. Chen Zhaopei and his uncle Chen Fa-ke established a martial arts school and endeavored to bring this lawlessness under control. The number of students who came to them increased rapidly, and the number of bandits decreased significantly.

In 1928 Chen Zhaopei was invited to Beijing by the famous "Tong Ren Tang" (Le brothers). Tong Ren Tang was a pharmacy that had been established at the beginning of the Qing dynasty and had prospered with thirty-four branches throughout China. With the fall of the Qing dynasty and the subsequent unrest in

China, Tong Ren Tang in Beijing was often raided or extorted for money. The Le brothers decided to engage a good martial artist in order to solve this problem. The store's accountant, who happened to come from Henan Province, recommended Chen Zhaopei.

Although Chen Zhaopei did not have many years of formal education (due to poverty), he was an upright and thoughtful man. He was aware that it would not be easy to set up as a martial artist without offending other schools and having to face many challenges. During his early days in Beijing he often disguised himself as a street vendor in order to observe other martial arts schools. Many times he was driven to protect the weak against the bullies of the area.

During this time he met a famous scholar, Li Qinlin, who was also from Henan. In his enthusiasm to meet someone from his home province, as well as his delight at Chen style Taijiquan being seen in Beijing at last, Li wrote an article that was published in the *Beijing Times* Newspaper. Beijing up until then had only witnessed Yang style Taijiquan. Li had often exalted the power and beauty of Chen style—the style that Yang Taiji had evolved from—but felt that he had not been able to convince many. In the article Li wrote about the merits of Chen style Taijiquan, he compared it to the popular martial arts around, stating that only in Chen style could one find the combination of strong and fast with relaxed and slow movement. He wrote about how it is beneficial for health as well as self-defense and pointed out the shortcomings of the other systems. Past Chen masters were described: Chen Wangting, Chen Changxing, Chen Genyun, Chen Zhongxin, Chen Yanxi, etc. The article ended with an invitation for those who had not experienced Chen style Taijiquan to "try it out," as a very skilled Chen descendent had arrived in Beijing.

The article, though well intentioned, brought problems for Chen Zhaopei. Other schools saw it as a challenge to their systems. After fighting off an isolated incident when one of the neighborhood bullies came to the pharmacy to test him out, Chen was urged to set up a *lei-tai* (martial podium) in Xuan Wu

Men (one of the many gates to Beijing) for the purpose of accepting all challenges.

In this manner, Chen Zhaopei took challenges for seventeen days, fighting over two hundred people in total. Some came to the podium alone, but mostly in threes and fives. Chen emerged undefeated and made friends of many martial artists from different schools. This was because he was magnanimous in victory and invariably showed his superiority without humiliating his opponents.

Chen Zhaopei's reputation spread far and wide after the *lei-tai*, and many invitations poured in requesting Chen's instruction. Invitations came from the Beijing government, Zhao Yang University, and the University of Beijing. A martial arts school was set up in readiness for Chen to commence teaching. Soon after this, however, Chen received an invitation from Wei Daoming, the mayor of Nanjing, to be a coach at the famous Central Martial Arts Institute.

Chen Zhaopei's new students were disconsolate on hearing that their newly found master was to leave. Seeing their disappointment, he thought for a while and then suggested a solution. He would invite his third uncle, Chen Fa-ke, whose "skill was ten times greater than his own," to teach them. With this, he sent a messenger back to the village to fetch him.

Chen Zhaopei went to Nanjing in 1930 and by 1933 had been elevated to the position of National Judge. In 1937, Nanjing fell into the hands of the Japanese, and Chen, unwilling to serve under the enemy, left the city. The subsequent years saw him involved in the resistance movement, as well as teaching the family system in various places such as Luoyang, Xian, etc.

In 1958 Chen Zhaopei, on a visit to Chenjiagou, became concerned about the state of Taijiquan in its birthplace. There was hardly anyone left in the village who was proficient in the art, and the younger generation was not being developed. This dire situation had arisen as a result of circumstances outside the control of the population. Natural disasters struck the area one after anoth-

FIGURE 7.6
David Gaffney in front
of monument for
Chen Zhaopei

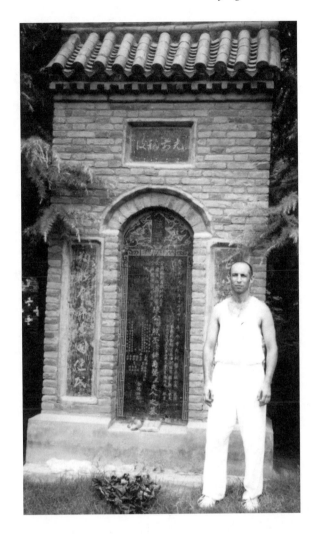

er. First there was flood, then drought, and finally locust infesta-
tion. For the villagers who relied almost exclusively upon agricul-
ture for their livelihood, survival became almost impossible. For a
countryside that was already far from wealthy, these disasters were
catastrophic. The younger and stronger people left the village in
order to seek their future in other provinces. The old generation
with skill soon left to teach their skills elsewhere. Very quickly Taiji
practice became less and less common. The numerous training
halls fell into disrepair, weapons racks were covered in dust, and

the weapons themselves became rusty from lack of use.

This was how Chen Zhaopei found the village on his return visit. He vowed to revive the practice of Taijiquan and develop a new generation of skilled practitioners. Chen took early retirement from his employment and used his own savings to set up a school in Chenjiagou.

The new generation of Taiji exponents was subsequently produced. Among them are the present four "Buddha's Warrior Attendants" or "Four Tigers," Chen Xiaowang, Chen Zhenglei, Zhu Tiancai and Wang Xian.

The road to success was not easy for Chen Zhaopei. During the Cultural Revolution (1966-1976), Chen was persecuted, sometimes severely, for practicing and propagating a traditional art. He was forced to endure public humiliation by wearing a dunce's hat as he was paraded through the streets. Training had to be carried out in secret, mostly at night. Chen Zhenglei mentioned an occasion when Chen Zhaopei waited up half the night, but nobody turned up for fear of reprisals. To work off his despair, he took out his sword and wielded it until he was drenched with sweat and totally exhausted.

In order to find a way around the dangers associated with practicing Taiji, Chen changed the traditional names of the forms into communist slogans, singing out loudly as he performed each posture. For example, the movement "Buddha's Warrior Attendant Pounds Mortar" was changed to "Chairman Mao Pounds Mortar." People thought that the old man had gone mad. Chen Zhaopei said:

> If they say I'm mad then I'm mad;
> If they say I'm insane then I'm insane;
> Why do I do these mad insane things?
> It's a determination to nurture future generations.

Towards the end of the dark period of the Cultural Revolution, Chairman Mao happened to mention the practice of Taijiquan in one of his speeches, thus giving endorsement to its practice. Chen Zhaopei sought Chen Zhenglei out with a crumpled newspaper that covered the speech, tears streaming down his face, to tell him the good news.

Things eased gradually, and public Taiji practice began again. Chen Zhaopei's book *Chen Shi Taijiquan Hai Ceng* was written during this time as a contribution to the state and to the art of Taijiquan. In 1972, Chenjiagou was allowed to participate in a province-level martial arts competition. Chen Zhaopei worked tirelessly in preparation for this event. Many difficult maneuvers and low postures had to be demonstrated. The training place was a mile away and Chen, who was nearly eighty years of age, walked the distance each day for nearly three months, enduring swollen, painful feet. When the competition was over, the team was selected to represent the province for the national competition. Chen's health finally succumbed and he was hospitalized. Against medical advice, he continued to actively train the team upon being discharged. This, however, was too much for his frail state and he died four days later. To this day, Chen Zhaopei is remembered for single-handedly reviving Taijiquan practice in the Chen Village and for his dedication to the family art.

Martial Virtue *(Wu-De)*

China has a history of several thousand years that places great emphasis on traditions and ceremonies. As early as the Spring and Autumn Period, Confucius (551–479 B.C.) realized the importance of etiquette and morals in maintaining harmony and order and thus keeping society together. He spent a lifetime promoting it. The ideal scholarly virtue was defined by the sixth century B.C., which included benevolence, gentleness and loyalty.

Martial arts require rigorous physical training that brings about fitness and self-defense skill. However, to reach higher levels, mental and character development must accompany physical skill, as it is believed that without moral character, the real essence of *wushu* (in this context, martial skill) will not be discovered by the practitioner. The proper development of character and spirit, therefore, is considered as important as physical attributes, and a code of ethics has been developed to foster the cultivation and refinement of character and personality. It is a self-regulatory practice among the martial community, as *wu* (martial skill) without the *de* (virtue) allows the practitioner to use his skill in a bad way. *Wu-de* embodies the five morals of Sun Zi's *The Art of War*: Wisdom, Loyalty, Benevolence, Courage, and Integrity.

Chen family Taijiquan has maintained a strict code of ethics throughout the generations. This is given as one of the reasons why the art was kept within the family and why the skill was not widespread in the past. Demands on the students were strict and without compromise. Before imparting any knowledge, a teacher had to carefully ascertain the character and ability of the student. A mistake could prove dangerous both for himself and the community. So it was when Chen Changxing taught Chen Taiji skill to Yang Luchan only after many years of observation.

In order to learn Taiji well, the first requirements must be diligence and perseverance. Taiji classics state: *"Without perseverance there can be no gain"* and *"Learning Taiji is like rowing a boat against the flow of water; if you do not go forward, you will drift back."* In order to glimpse the full wonder of Taiji and to attain a high level of skill, one must possess a will to carry on despite hardship, setbacks, frustration and boredom. From the beginning, students must be willing to commit themselves to a long-term goal and be patient during the process of achieving that goal. The process of learning takes time, and the necessary length of time must be allowed to understand the content of the teaching. One will not succeed if focus is only on the final product.

A fundamental moral obligation demanded of all martial practitioners is benevolence. Taijiquan classics say: *"Proficiency in Taijiquan should not lead to arrogance as arrogance invites trouble; one should not be arrogant with the hands or with the speech."* Therefore, do not initiate a fight and do not covet (person, possession or nation). Instead, the first consideration should be to stop a fight and keep the peace. Treat peers with respect and be magnanimous. Relationships should be based on interaction and respect, not dominance or submission. Do not challenge the arrogant and do not argue with the ignorant. Avoiding a situation should be the first course of action. However, in an unavoidable situation, defend oneself. Even then, show restraint by stopping when one has the upper hand. When faced with a real enemy, however, be brave and courageous and do not show mercy. Both the physical and mental aspects of martial arts then move into play, united in action.

Humility and honesty are important aspects of *de*. Humility ensures open-mindedness and eagerness to learn. Always demand improvement of oneself and have keen motivation for practice. Taijiquan classics say that *"learning quan also teaches humility. A lack of humility impedes progress."* Therefore, one should avoid excessive pride and over-confidence. During exchange of skill, give due respect to those with higher abilities and do not display jealousy and envy. Show consideration to those of lesser skill and do not treat them with disdain and insults. The famous seventeenth-generation master Chen Fa-ke was renowned for his respect and consideration for others, students and contemporaries alike, always magnanimous in victory. He believed that one's skill is recognized and respected not by force, but by heartfelt conviction of one's ability.

Honesty is not just being honest in one's dealings with others, but also the acceptance of one's own limitations and shortcomings. It takes strength and courage to deal with one's own weaknesses. There should be a constant striving for improvement. Over-confidence makes a person stop learning, as he is too easily satisfied with his accomplishments. There must be a beginner's mentality throughout the pursuit for the highest possible goal.

Taijiquan classics used the terms honor and respect in two contexts. The first is to honor and respect your teacher, and the second is for your body. *"Do not neglect your teacher and do not neglect your body. If your heart is not mindful, how can you learn your skill?"* Traditionally the Chinese allocated hierarchy as Heaven, Earth,

Ruler, Parents, and Teacher. This emphasizes the importance of a teacher's position in society. When learning from a traditional Chinese teacher, once you have ascertained that he is the one to trust and respect, it may be helpful to know, acknowledge and accept this teacher-student relationship. The relationship may require the student not to judge what is right or wrong, which does not mean that the student should just follow blindly. It is sometimes a matter of asking too many questions too soon, demanding complex knowledge before even the basics are practiced or understood. One should guard against projecting ahead for movements and technique without first going through the proper training sequence.

"Do not neglect your body" means do not forget to practice your *quan* to the best of your ability. The body should not be abused but should be kept healthy and in its optimum condition.

Chen Family Ancestral Law *(Men Gui)*

The Chen Family has its own essential rules for those who have taken up the practice of Chen style Taijiquan. They comprise the three main areas that are deemed crucial to one's development, not only of martial skill but spiritual growth.

The Twelve Characters

1. Decorous

2. Respectful

3. Just

4. Upright

5. Kind

6. Noble

7. Magnanimous

8. Courageous

9. Honest

10. Trustworthy

11. Sincere

12. Virtuous

The Twenty Disciplines

1. Do not bully others.

2. Do not oppress the weak.

3. Do not be a coward; help those in peril.

4. Do not engage in unlawful acts.

5. Do not use skill for immoral acts.

6. Do not be arrogant.

7. Do not sell/exhibit skill indiscriminately.

8. Do not join illicit gangs.

9. Do not waste time in idleness.

10. Do not be conceited and boastful.

11. Do not compete with the arrogant.

12. Do not argue with the ignorant.

13. Do not be influenced by worldly possessions.

14. Do not seek undeserved wealth.

15. Do not indulge in alcohol and lust.

16. Do not be in public or personal debt.

17. Do not obstruct public or personal efforts.

18. Do not hunger for power and position.

19. Do not be a traitor.

20. Do not neglect your training or waste your skill.

The Twelve Vices

1. Deviance

2. Evil

3. Undependability

4. Cunning

5. Recklessness

6. Duplicity

7. Exaggeration

8. Immorality

9. Deceit

10. Dishonesty

11. Arrogance

12. Cruelty

"A decent and upright person learns the *quan* in order to keep his body healthy and strong, and to defend himself—this is the core teaching of the Chen Family."

"The deviant, unscrupulous person learns the *quan* in order to intimidate and harm others—this is absolutely forbidden by the Chen Family."

Bibliography

Chen Xiaowang, *Chen Style Taijiquan Transmitted Through Generations*.
  People's Sports Publishing Beijing (1990).
Chen Xin, *Illustrated Explanation of Chen Family Taijiquan*. Shanghai Bookstore
  (1986).
Chen Zhenglei, *A Compendium of Taijiquan Boxing and Weapons*
  (3 Volumes). Higher Education Press, Beijing (1992).
Chen Zhenglei, *The Art of Chen Family Taijiquan*. Technical Sports
  Publications, Shanxi (1999).
Diepersloot, Jan, *Warriors of Stillness: Meditative Traditions in the Chinese Martial
  Arts*. Vol. I. Walnut Creek, CA, Center for Healing and the Arts
  (1995).
Feng Zhiqiang, *Entering the Door of Chen Style Taijiquan*. People's Sports
  Publishing, Beijing (1993).
Feng Zhiqiang, Feng Dabiao, Chen Xiaowang, *Chen Style Taijiquan*.
  Morning Glory Publishers, Beijing (1988).
Gu Liuxin, Shen Jiazheng, *Chen Style Taijiquan*. People's Sports Publishing,
  Beijing (1994).
Gu Liuxin, *The Origin, Evolution and Development of Shadow Boxing*. Peoples
  Sports Publishing, Beijing (1988).
Henning, Stanley E., Ignorance, Legend and Taijiquan in *Journal of Chen
  Style Taijiquan*. Research Association of Hawaii, Vol. 2,
  No. 3.
History of China (4 Volumes). Haiyen Publications (2000).
Hu Bing, *A Brief Introduction to the Science of Breathing Exercise*. Hai Feng
  Publishing, Hong Kong (1982).

Hu Zhaoyun, ed., *Chinese Qigong*. Publishing House of Shanghai College of Traditional Chinese Medicine (1988).

I Ching: The Classic Chinese Oracle of Change. Trans. Rudolf Ritsema & Stephen Karchen. Element Books UK (1994).

Journal of Asian Martial Arts. Erie, PA: Via Media Publishing.

Lao Tsu, *Tao Te Ching*. Trans. Gia Fu Feng & Jane English. Wildwood House Ltd., England (1973).

Ma Hong, *Chen Style Taijiquan Method and Theory*. Beijing Sports University Press (1998).

Schipper, Kristofer, *The Taoist Body*. Pelanduk Publications, Malaysia (1996).

Seidel, Anna, "A Taoist Immortal of the Ming Dynasty: Chang San-Feng" in *W.T. de Bary & The Conference on Ming Thought*. New York: Columbia University Press (1970).

Sun Zi, *The Art of War*. Trans. Lo Ziye. Beijing University Press (1995).

Tai Chi Magazine. Wayfarer Publications, Los Angeles.

Tang Hao, *Shaolin-Wudang Research*. Unicorn Press, Hong Kong (1968).

The Complete Book of Taijiquan. People's Sports Publishing, Beijing (1995).

The Location of Acupoints: State Standard of the People's Republic of China. Foreign Language Press, Beijing (1990).

Xu Longhou, *Illustrated Explanations of Taijiquan Forms*. Zhonghuo Wushu Press, Taipei (1921).

Xu Zhedong, *Correct Approach Towards and Recognition of False Aspects of Taijiquan Manuals*. Zhenshan Mei Press, Taipei (1965).

Zhao Ganjie, *Heroic Tales of Chen Family Taijiquan*. Zhongzhou Gu Ji Publications (1997).

Zhu Tiancai, *Authentic Chenjiagou Taijiquan*. Percetaken Turbo Sdn. Bhd., Malaysia (1994).

Zhu Tiancai, Various papers and articles.

Index

R

Red Spear Gang, 205
Ren mai (conception channel), 14,
62, 63, 102
rou (softness), 35, 73–74, 93,
112, 137

S

san shou, 112
Shaolin boxing, 12, 17, 28, 29,
141
Shaolin Temple, 12
shen, 54, 102, 104, 112, 113
Shen Jiazheng, 153
Shenfa, 53
shoufa (hand techniques), 78
shun-chan, 50, 51, 66, 76,
108–109, 116, 166
silk-reeling energy—see *chan ssu
jing*
si xiang, 122
single-movement exercises, 6,
135–137
Small Heavenly Circulation, 102
song, 35, 60, 75, 151
spear *(qiang)*, 16, 44, 91, 171,
181–186
spring and autumn broadsword
(guan dao), 44, 171, 186–190,
Spring and Autumn Period, 211
standing pole, 6, 45, 66, 103,
106–108, 111, 143
Sun Jianyun, 26
Sun Lutang, 26
Sun style Taijiquan, 26
Sun Zi, 163, 166, 212
sword *(jian)*, 22, 44, 91, 171,
172–178, 179, 192, 197, 210

T

taiji tu, 32
taiji-ball, 143, 145–146
taiji-bang (ruler), 143, 146–147
Tang Hao, 27, 29, 30, 181, 201
taolu—see forms
"Three Cleansings of
Huaiqing," 9
"three internal connections,"
74, 86
"three external connections,"
76, 86
Three Kingdoms Period, 187
Tien Moer, 9
tu-na, 2–3, 14, 33, 81

W

Wang Maozhai, 24
Wang Peisheng, 24
Wang Xian, 22, 210
weapons, 6, 44, 80, 82, 91, 92,
103, 171–190, 196, 199,
209–210
Weizhong, 66, 99
wu-de (martial virtue), 211–214
Wu (Hao) style Taijiquan, 24, 25
Wu Jianquan, 23, 24
Wu Kongcho, 165
Wu style Taijiquan, 23, 24, 165
Wu Yinghwa, 24
Wu Yuxiang, 24
wuji, 32, 71, 81, 100, 104, 121,
123
wu-wei, 37

David Gaffney
Davidine Siaw-Voon Sim
Chenjiagou Taijiquan GB
14 Clifton Ave, Culcheth,
Warrington WA3 4PD
United Kingdom